FACTS AND COMPARISONS

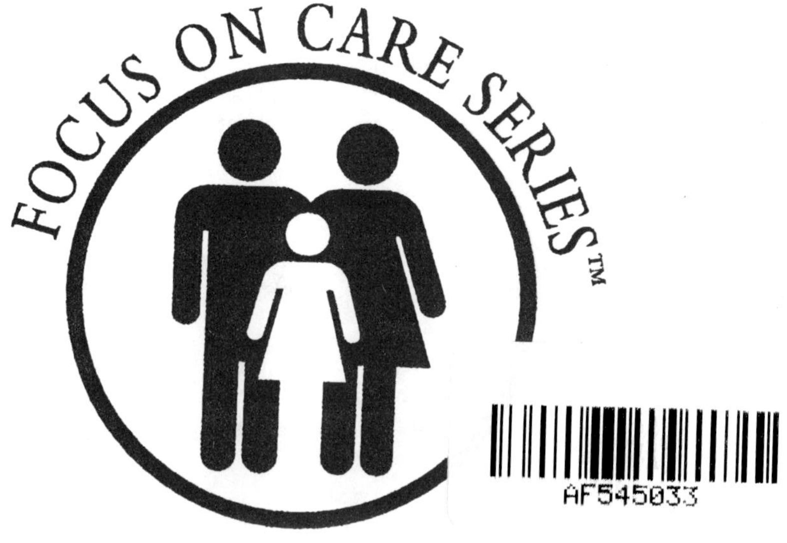

Immunization Delivery: A Complete Guide

A Community Health Handbook

The author and publisher took care to assure that uses, warnings, doses, and schedules are correct and agree with standards generally accepted at the time of publication. Readers are cautioned to apply their own judgment in all health-care decisions.

This information is advisory only and does not replace sound clinical judgment or individualized patient care. Facts and Comparisons, Inc., and the authors disclaim all warranties, expressed or implied, including any warranty as to the quality, accuracy, or suitability of this information for any particular purpose. Listing of specific products is a sign only of availability on the market and is not an endorsement or recommendation.

Suggested Citation:
Grabenstein JD. *Immunization Delivery: A Complete Guide.* St. Louis: Facts and Comparisons, 1997:(inclusive pages).

ISBN 1-57439-020-1

Printed in the United States of America

Address correspondence to the author via the publisher.

Immunization Delivery: A Complete Guide
Published by Facts and Comparisons
a **Wolters Kluwer** Company
111 West Port Plaza, Suite 300
St. Louis, MO 63146-3098
Customer Service 800-223-0554
314-878-2515
FAX 314-878-5563

Immunization Delivery: A Complete Guide

John D. Grabenstein, MS Pharm, EdM, FASHP, FRSH

Vincent J. Parker	President
Steven K. Hebel, RPh	Publisher, Pharmacy
Teri H. Burnham	Project Editor
Julie A. Scott	Market Development Coordinator
Sara L. Schweain	Assistant Editor
Renée M. Short	Assistant Editor
Jennifer K. Walsh	Composition Specialist

Facts and Comparisons
St. Louis
A **Wolters Kluwer** Company

DEDICATION

To my wonderful wife, Laurie Ann, with love and thanks;
to Emily, to Andrea, and to Erica, with hope;
and to Mom & Dad, with love and thanks.
[Erica's contribution to this book at age 5 months:
gttttttbvvb tvgdfxdgxgdtvdv0']

ACKNOWLEDGEMENTS

It is not possible to complete any work of this size alone. I am indebted to many people, most notably my family. My teachers in Cumberland, Pittsburgh, Bremerhaven, Chapel Hill, and throughout the Army opened my eyes to the wonders of the world and the miracles of science. The professionals at Facts and Comparisons are both colleagues and friends. To these and many more people, I are very grateful.

J.D.G.

About the Author: John D. Grabenstein, MS Pharm, EdM, FASHP, FRSH, is a clinical pharmacist with the United States Army Medical Department. He was spent over 15 years studying immunology, epidemiology and vaccine advocacy. The author wrote this book in his private capacity. No official support or endorsement by the US Department of the Army or Department of Defense is intended, nor should it be inferred.

Table of Contents

Chapter 1 - Introduction: Focus on Prevention 1
Chapter 2 - Too Many Deaths, Too Much Disease: The Vaccine-Preventable Diseases 7
- Influenza & Pneumonia 8
- Hepatitis B 11
- "Childhood" Diseases 13
  - Measles 13
  - Mumps 14
  - Rubella 14
  - Varicella 15
  - Diphtheria 16
  - Tetanus 16
  - Pertussis 17
  - Poliomyelitis 18
  - *Haemophilus influenzae* type b 19
  - "Childhood" Disease Among Adolescents and Adults 20
- Vaccine Advice Based on Age 21
- Vaccine Advice Based on Personal Factors 23
- Diseases & Diagnoses of People Needing Vaccines 25
- Medications of People Needing Vaccines 26

Chapter 3 - The Science of Vaccinology: How Vaccines & Antibodies Work 29
- Vaccines Are Drugs 29
- Differential Pharmacology 29
  - Cellular vs Humoral Immunity 29
  - Active vs Passive Immunity 30
  - Primary vs Booster Responses 31
  - Disease vs Infection 31
  - Local vs Circulating Antibodies 31
  - Killed vs Live Vaccines 32
  - Toxoids vs Vaccines 32
  - Polysaccharide vs Proteinaceous Vaccines 33
  - Human vs Animal Antibodies 33
  - Drug Interactions 34
- Differential Pharmaceutics 34
  - Subunit vs Whole Vaccines 34
  - Solutions vs Suspensions 35
  - Standard vs Hyperimmune Antibodies 35
  - Production Methods 36
  - Preferred vs Inadequate Diluents 37
- Differential Utilization 38

Chapter 4 - Making Vaccine Decisions 43
Finding Those Who Need Vaccines 43
How To Motivate Vaccine Candidates 45
Model of Health Behavior 45
Interviewing People About Immunizations 46
Phase I: Assessment 46
Phase II: Decision-Making 54
Phase III: Education & Consent 57
Phase IV: Confirmation 60
Chapter 5 - Special Situations 65
Customizing Immunization Plans 65
Pregnancy 65
Breast-Feeding 67
Issues of Age 67
International Travel 67
Underlying Disease 68
Weakened Immune Systems 68
Immune Response 69
Infection Risk 70
Vaccines for People Infected with HIV 71
Live Bacterial or Viral Vaccines 71
Inactivated Vaccines or Toxoids 71
Safety of Immunizing HIV-Infected People 73
Chapter 6 - Immunization Administration 77
Administration Guidelines 79
Choosing a Route 84
Emergency Plans 83
Response to a Systemic Reaction 84
Epinephrine Doses 85
Diphenhydramine Doses 86
Other Urgent Situations 87
Visit Sketches 89
Chapter 7 - Immunization Documentation 93
Vaccine Records for Clinicians 94
Annotated Screening Form for Vaccines & Tuberculin Tests 95
Informed-Consent Documents 103
Vaccine Records for Patients 103
Lost Records 104
Synthesis 104

Chapter 8 - Administrative Issues ... 107
Facility Design ... 107
Marketing and Management Issues ... 107
Obtaining Compensation ... 108
Medicare Reimbursement for Immunization ... 108
Questions and Answers About Medicare's Influenza Vaccination Benefit ... 112
Chapter 9 - Legal & Liability Issues ... 123
Professional Liability ... 123
Protections Under State Law ... 124
Business Liability ... 125
Liability for Administering Vaccines ... 125
Risk Reduction ... 128
Failing to Vaccinate ... 128
Compensation for Vaccine Injury ... 128
Adjudication ... 130
Chapter 10 - Pharmacy's Role in Immunization Delivery ... 135
Pharmacy's Unique Contributions ... 135
What Pharmacists Have Accomplished To Date ... 137
Pharmacists as Vaccine Leaders ... 140
Roles for Community Pharmacists ... 141
Roles for Hospital Pharmacists ... 141
Roles for Nursing-Home Consultants ... 142
Model Immunization Practices ... 142
Unique Legal Issues ... 143
Chapter 11 - Nursing's Role in Immunization Delivery ... 147
Nursing's Unique Contributions ... 147
Nurses as Vaccine Leaders ... 147
Roles for Hospital Nurses ... 148
Roles in Nursing Homes ... 149
Unique Legal Issues ... 150
Chapter 12 - Medicine's Role in Immunization Delivery ... 153
Maximize Prevention in Your Practice ... 153
Remove Barriers to Immunization ... 153
Know Valid Contraindications ... 154
Educate Patients ... 154
Educate Your Community ... 154
Help Hospitals Participate ... 154
Help Nursing Homes Participate ... 155
Use Free Vaccine ... 155
Assessment & Feedback ... 155

Chapter 13 - Getting Started 159
Four Steps 159
Community Catalysts 160
Eliminate Missed Opportunities 161
Key Questions To Help Advocates Get Started 162
Annex A - Advocacy Ideas 165
Annex B - Resources Available 169
Annex C - Vaccine Adverse Event Reporting System (VAERS) and MedWatch 175
Annex D - Hypersensitivities to Vaccine Components 179
Index 183

CHAPTER 1

Introduction: Focus on Prevention

Are you doing all you can to keep your patients healthy? What role do you take in the battle to stop preventable infections? Have you recommended an immunization to anyone lately?

This book is a resource for healthcare professionals who are starting or expanding their clinical services to deliver immunizations. The pages are full of facts, figures and helpful ideas to keep patients healthy.

Too many of America's children are incompletely protected from serious diseases. Even worse, nearly 100,000 American adults die each year because of lack in immunizations. Tens of millions of Americans are vulnerable to disability and fatal infections that can be prevented if you act. Most of these people have ready access to a healthcare professional: Their family pharmacist, nurse or physician.[1-4]

Immunization advocacy is gathering momentum. See how you and your colleagues can protect your community.

Many people talk about the value of prevention, but few are blending prevention activities into their everyday practice. You can be a forward-thinking professional of the 21st century right now if you take responsibility for keeping the families in your practice healthy.[5-6]

This book contains dozens of ways to become a vaccine advocate. Read on: You will find many good ideas. More important, you will see why focusing on immunization delivery is vital.

Prevention Is Different

If you think vaccines are just another set of drugs in your refrigerator or just an expense line in your budget, you are missing the point. Advocacy is about reaching out to patients in need, not waiting for someone to ask for the vaccine. If vaccines expire in your refrigerator – unused, wasted – it is your practice's fault for not advocating their use sufficiently. Rarely is there a valid reason for a vaccine's potency to expire.[7]

Practices are inanimate. It is not right to blame a practice for failing to do something. Rather, it is pharmacists, nurses and physicians who make up these practices. It is they who act or fail to act to keep people healthy. By assertive vaccine advocacy, we can avert death itself. Whether you are director of the practice, the newest staff member, a technician or a student, you are a medication specialist who influences colleagues and patients.

By remaining silent you tolerate people being inactive and vulnerable. By calling for increased delivery of immunizations, you influence people toward taking a preventive action. You can have a positive influence.

Despite reports of spot shortages, enough influenza vaccine is returned to manufacturers each year to vaccinate millions of people. Although pneumococcal vaccines have been available since 1977, less than a quarter of the people at risk are immunized. If we have the will, the vast majority of 50,000 to 80,000 deaths and countless human misery can be prevented.

Prevention is fundamentally different from therapy. With therapy, a sick person appears in front of you. You then fix or mitigate his or her health problem. Prevention requires the vision to foresee problems and avert them in people who do not yet have symptoms. Seeing the sick person is the stimulus in therapy.

Think about your children, your spouse, your parents, your family: Would you act to keep them healthy? Do the same for the patients you care for in your practice. It takes time and energy to brush teeth, buy insurance, choose healthy diets, fasten seat belts, get medical and dental check-ups, select cars with air bags, etc. Do the same with vaccines.

If you are ready to act to keep your patients healthy, read on. You may have seen the bumper sticker that urges, "Think Globally, Act Locally." Some people around you will die or suffer if you do not act. The people who depend on you for care also depend on you for prevention. Prevent all the disease you can, then treat the rest.

The Problem and the Solution

The death toll and illness from vaccine-preventable diseases will be discussed in the following chapter. Although a sizeable allotment of resources is, and needs to be, devoted to immunizing children, 400 adults die from a vaccine-preventable disease for each child who dies of one.[1-4]

Vaccine-preventable deaths exceed the fatalities from 100 jumbo jets crashing each year. Imagine the furor if two big jets crashed each week. That is how many people die needlessly from influenza and pneumonia.

Time after time, demonstration projects and publications show that most people follow the advice of pharmacists, nurses and physicians who recommend immunizations. Typically, 50% to 75% or more get vaccinated if a professional they trust recommends a vaccine to them.[8-11]

We know that kids need their shots. What about adults? People just like you have found many clever ways to identify patients at the highest risk of disease, especially for influenza and pneumococcal disease. The people with diabetes who need protection are recorded in medical and prescription databases with that diagnosis or as users of insulin or oral hypoglycemic agents.[8-9,12] People with serious respiratory disease who need to be vaccinated are recorded as chronic users of beta-adrenergic agonists, inhaled steroids, theophylline and the like. You will find patients with chronic cardiovascular disease from records of digoxin, warfarin, nitroglycerin and many other cardiovascular drugs. Children on chronic aspirin therapy are at risk of Reye's syndrome if they get a viral infection. An influenza vaccine will reduce that risk. People ≥ 65 years of age also need to be vaccinated.

Prescription and medical databases can be used to produce customized letters to people, warning them of their infection risk and motivating them to be vaccinated. Veterinarians send postcards to their patients who need immunizations; Why don't you? Or program your computer to do it.

Vaccine Advocacy

The great thing about vaccine advocacy is that you can choose for yourself: Wade in or jump in head first. Vaccine advocacy takes little extra time beyond your current activities. Just blend vaccine advocacy into your daily routine. You will find specific ideas throughout this book.

- Level 1: If you want to start slowly while juggling other responsibilities, be a motivator. This involves teaching, warning, advising, alerting, informing, answering questions, enlightening and reaching out. Some of these activities are passive; others are more active.
- Level 2: If you are ready for a more vibrant, assertive role, be a facilitator. Work with your colleagues to identify people needing vaccines. Consider admissions, discharges, emergency visits, diagnoses, prescriptions, clinical procedures, critical pathways, utilization review, discharge planning or mass screening.
- Level 3: If you want to be fully involved in the immunization outcome itself, get your practice ready and administer vaccinations yourself. If you already immunize, look around to see if vulnerable patients are slipping through cracks and leaving unprotected.

So many people need immunizations; so many are susceptible to vaccine-preventable diseases that activities at any of the three levels will be a big help to your community.

How to Use This Book

You can use *Immunization Delivery: A Complete Guide* in several ways. You can read it cover to cover; although it would be most gratifying to the author, it may not be best suited to your purposes.

Specific chapters or annexes may hold the answers to your most urgent questions about immunization delivery. The detailed table of contents and index will help you find the information you want, fast. Take a glance at them to help find your way around.

If you want to find out which vaccines a patient needs, use chapter two on "Too Many Deaths, Too Much Disease" with its helpful tables. These sections identify who needs which vaccine.

There are separate chapters on the science of vaccines, the human factors about decision-making, special considerations regarding the vaccinee's health status, all the forms of documentation of immunizations and administrative and legal issues. One chapter is dedicated to each of the health professions most involved with vaccines: Pharmacists, nurses and physicians. You will probably want to read your profession's chapter first, but there may be ideas you can profit from in the other chapters as well.

Paradoxically, the last chapter is entitled "Getting Started." If you are already well underway as a vaccine advocate, think of this chapter as hitting the accelerator. Next, check out the annexes, especially the ones on resources, tools, standards and the like. The other annexes include all the helpful information we could assemble to boost your immunization practice. Once your practice is at full speed, help coach a colleague into becoming a vaccine advocate.

How to Become an Advocate

Becoming a vaccine advocate or an immunizer is not particularly difficult, but it does require preparation. To get started, learn the issues, gather information and talk to vaccine experts in your practice site or your community. Seek partners in your county and among your colleagues. Expert courses on immunizations are available from the Centers for Disease Control & Prevention (CDC), often via video telecourses at local health departments or colleges. Volunteering briefly with county health clinics also may be helpful. Educate yourself, one step at a time by using resources readily available to you.

A separate chapter on "Getting Started" will give you many details, but the general principles on how to begin vaccine advocacy are:

1.) Decide which level of immunization advocacy you will adopt. Gather information about immunizations in your institution or your community (eg, local health clinic). Ask who, what, when, where, how much, how often? Develop a plan that meets the needs of the people around you. Remember, influenza and pneumonia account for the most deaths.
2.) Prepare your practice and your staff. Discuss the need for vaccines. Do whatever it takes in preparing to implement your plan. For example, prepare handouts to send to your patients or to dispense with each prescription. Organize your persuasive message to best motivate your target audience.
3.) Implement your program. For example, send notices to the people most at risk. Answer questions from patients. Brag about the good things you have done. Have your public relations office issue a press release or call the local news media.
4.) Keep up the good work. Be an advocate all year long. Use whatever you did this year as a basis for doing even more next year.

Every Action Produces Results

Just about anything you do in vaccine advocacy will bear fruit in the form of better health, avoided disease and longer life.

"People Are Dying While Unused Vaccines Sit in Refrigerators"

If you saw that headline in your hometown newspaper or heard it on the evening news, how would you react? What would you tell the reporter who asked about your role? Would you say that it was not your fault, that nobody asked you for the vaccines? Would you contend that the deceased never asked to be vaccinated?[7]

People do not just walk in off the street and ask for digoxin or insulin, but we figure out who needs to be medicated and offer our expertise to them. All health professionals are responsible for keeping patients healthy. It may sound perverse, but I look forward to the day when failing to properly offer vaccinations is widely considered negligence. Proper immunization advocacy should be the standard of care in all practices.

People needing immunizations appear in clinics, hospitals, offices and pharmacies every day. They are patients, coworkers, family and friends.

Our grandparents dreaded that loved ones would be stricken with polio, diphtheria, smallpox, pertussis, measles, tetanus and similar plagues. Public swimming pools would close in the 1950s in the heat of the summer in a futile attempt to stop polio outbreaks from spreading. Using safe and effective vaccines means few people die of childhood diseases anymore.

Despite our successes against polio, diphtheria and the like, influenza and pneumonia take our elders from us far earlier than need be. We can stop that with vaccines.

American healthcare is not doing a good enough job getting vaccines to the right population. We can help bridge the gap and find the vulnerable people. Do we deserve new vaccines against other diseases if we cannot adequately deliver the ones we have?

Relative Cost-effectiveness

To keep things in perspective, the accompanying table shows a variety of cost-effective measures. Cost-effectiveness estimates depend on the cost of an intervention, the number of people who must be treated or tested to avert a problem, the benefit of the intervention and other factors.[13-16]

The first four entries show the amount of money Americans spend to gain a year of life from various technologies. The next three entries show cost savings resulting from immunizations delivered. The final entry reminds us that vaccines do not have to save money to be worthwhile. Avoiding disease and death has value to the individual and to society that is worth the money. America spends far more money on other diseases (eg, hypertension, high cholesterol) with a lesser return on investment (eg, cost per life-year saved).

Relative Cost-Effectiveness

Smoking-cessation therapy	$8,463 to gain 1 year of life
Renal dialysis	$46,249 to gain 1 year of life
Colestipol to lower cholesterol	$85,519 to gain 1 year of life
Coronary artery bypass graft (CABG) surgery	$113,087 to gain 1 year of life
Influenza vaccine	$117 saved per vaccinee
Measles-mumps-rubella vaccine	$12:1 savings ratio
Pneumococcal vaccine, high risk	$1.3:1 savings ratio
Pneumococcal vaccine for all	$2.3 cost for $1 spent

Need More Information?

We tried to include everything you might want to know about vaccine advocacy and delivery in this book. If we missed something you are interested in, write to us and let us know. We will try to include it with the next edition.

References

[1] Public Health Service, US Department of Health & Human Services. Immunization & Infectious Disease. In: *Healthy People 2000: National Health Promotion & Disease Prevention Objectives.* Washington, DC: Government Printing Office, 1991:511-28.

[2] Advisory Committee on Immunization Practices. General recommendations on immunization. *MMWR* 1994;43(RR-1):1-38.

[3] American College of Physicians. *Guide for Adult Immunization,* 3rd ed. Philadelphia: American College of Physicians, 1994.

[4] Peter G, ed. 1994 Red Book: Report of the Committee on Infectious Diseases, 23rd ed. Elk Grove Village, IL: American Academy of Pediatrics, 1994.

[5] Russell LB. *Is Prevention Better Than Cure?* Washington, DC: Brookings Institution, 1986.

[6] US Preventive Services Task Force. *Guide to Clinical Preventive Services,* 2nd ed. Baltimore: Williams & Wilkins, 1996.

[7] Grabenstein JD. Are vaccines expiring in your refrigerator? Become an advocate! *Hosp Pharm* 1996;31:1075-6,1081-2,1084,1086-8.

[8] Grabenstein JD, Hayton B. Pharmacoepidemiologic program for identifying patients in need of vaccination. *Am J Hosp Pharm* 1990;47:1774-80.

[9] Grabenstein JD, Hartzema AG, Guess HA, et al. Community pharmacists as immunization advocates: A clinical pharmacoepidemiologic experiment. *Internat J Pharm Pract* 1993;2:5-10.

[10] Spruill WJ, Cooper JW, Taylor WJR. Pharmacist-coordinated pneumonia and influenza vaccination program. *Am J Hosp Pharm* 1982;39:1904-6.

[11] Morton MR, Spruill WJ, Cooper JW. Pharmacist impact on pneumococcal vaccination rates in long-term-care facilities. *Am J Hosp Pharm* 1988;45:73 (letter).

[12] Grabenstein JD. *ImmunoFacts: Vaccines & Immunologic Drugs.* St. Louis: Facts and Comparisons, May 1997.

[13] Willems JS, Sanders CR. Cost-effectiveness and cost-benefit analyses of vaccines. *J Infect Dis* 1981;144:486-93.

[14] Weinstein MC. Economics of prevention: The costs of prevention. *J Gen Intern Med* 1990;5(Suppl):S89-92.

[15] van den Oever R, de Graeve D, Hepp B, et al. Pharmacoeconomics of immunization: A review. *PharmacoEconomics* 1993;3286-308.

[16] Sisk JE, Riegelman RK. Cost effectiveness of vaccination against pneumococcal pneumonia. *Ann Intern Med* 1986;104:79-86.

CHAPTER 2

Too Many Deaths, Too Much Disease: The Vaccine-Preventable Diseases

Early in the 1900s, the leading causes of death included smallpox and diphtheria. Diseases like measles, pertussis, rubella and polio caused terrific suffering as well. In the following years, vaccines against these and other infections were widely used to minimize the suffering and deaths.

Vaccines succeeded so well that many diseases have been forgotten. Forgotten, yes, but not gone. The microbes that cause these diseases are still around and will return if we let down our guard.

The following table shows how far disease levels have fallen since the adoption of vaccines.[1-5] Despite these successes, vaccine-preventable infections still harm and kill many Americans. That can be seen in the second table, showing the magnitude of needless losses from influenza, pneumococcal disease and hepatitis B.

Disease Control Through Immunization[1-5]

"Childhood" Disease	Peak Reported Cases	Minimum Reported Cases	Total 1995 Cases	1996 Provisional Case Total
Congenital rubella syndrome	≈20,000 in 1964-65	7 in 1995	6	2
Diphtheria	206,939 in 1921	0 in 1993	0	1
Haemophilus influenzae type b	≈20,000 in 1985	1,174 in 1993	1,180	1,078
Hepatitis B	a	a	10,167	b
Measles	894,134 in 1941	310 in 1995	310	494
Mumps	152,209 in 1968	906 in 1995	906	666
Pertussis	265,269 in 1934	1,010 in 1976	5,137	6,911
Polio, paralytic	21,269 in 1952	6 in 1995	6	1
Rubella	57,686 in 1969	128 in 1995	128	210
Tetanus (deaths)	1,560 in 1923	41 in 1995	41	28

a - Not reported.
b - Underreported to a far greater degree than other diseases listed.

Leading Causes of Vaccine-Preventable Infection[1-6]

	Infections per year, US	Deaths per year, US
Influenza A and B	25 to 50 million	10,000 to 40,000
Pneumococcal disease	≈555,000	40,000
Hepatitis B	150,000 to 200,000	5,000

Influenza and Pneumonia

Influenza and pneumonia are the sixth leading cause of death in the US. More alarming, the rate of death from these causes is rising, even after adjusting for the aging population. Influenza and pneumococcal pneumonia strike millions of people each year.[4,6-10]

Influenza

Influenza A and B lead to at least 10,000 to 40,000 deaths per year, about 80% among the elderly. The toll is even higher in epidemic years. For example, in 1991, some 77,000 influenza deaths were recorded. To compound the problem, influenza may precipitate other deaths that are attributed to cardiac, pulmonary or other causes. About 10% to 20% of the US population gets influenza each year.[11]

Influenza is characterized by an abrupt onset of fever, muscle ache, sore throat and nonproductive cough. Its complications include either a primary viral pneumonia or a secondary bacterial pneumonia. Influenza can lead to Reye's syndrome if aspirin is consumed by children after viral infection. Other complications include myocarditis or death. Fatalities occur in about one of every 1,000 to 2,000 cases.

America has finally reached the point of immunizing 60% of senior citizens against influenza, but that still leaves 40% vulnerable. Worse, only about 20% to 30% of younger people in high-risk groups are protected.[6]

A pandemic of influenza in 1918-19 killed 21 million, about 1% of the planet's global population. This was more than the death tolls of World War I and World War II combined. Lesser pandemics occurred around the world in 1932, 1957 and 1968. Scientists believe the next influenza pandemic is overdue. More than 20,000 excess deaths resulted from each of 10 influenza epidemics from 1972 to 1991. More than 40,000 deaths occurred in each of three epidemics during that interval. These epidemics cost well over $12 billion in direct medical and indirect societal costs.[11-12]

Influenza viruses change surface antigens much more quickly than other microbes. These changes make it hard for the body to defend itself against influenza. Two kinds of antigenic changes are recognized: Antigenic drift and antigenic shift. Antigenic drift, the more common type, involves minor changes in antigenic characteristics. This drift happens constantly and is associated with epidemics if differences are big enough. It is antigenic drift that necessitates annual changes in influenza vaccine formulations. Antigenic shift occurs less often and consists of major changes sufficient to warrant designation of a new subtype. Because humans have not been previously exposed to the new antigenic configuration, another influenza pandemic can be expected.

To increase the likelihood of vaccine efficacy, three viral types are included in each dose of vaccine: Type A (subtype H1N1), type A (subtype H3N2), and type B. Each spring, influenza experts predict which viral strains of those three types will be circulating in the following autumn. Then vaccine manufacturers can begin growing those viruses in fertilized chicken eggs. Each egg yields enough virus for only one or two doses of vaccine, so millions of fertilized eggs are required for each year's batches of influenza vaccine. Viral strain predictions over the last decade have been accurate.

Most doses of influenza vaccine are given between October and December each year. This allows enough time for vaccine recipients to respond to the vaccine by producing antibodies before epidemics begin. Influenza disease peaks between December and March in most places, a little earlier in Alaska. The most value comes by vaccinating early, but vaccination should continue throughout the influenza season, even into March, as additional unprotected people at risk are identified.

Two kinds of influenza A and B vaccine are manufactured. Both contain inactivated viruses, either in whole- or split-virus form. The split-virus or split-virion form produces fewer mild fevers in children and is preferred in that group. The two kinds have comparable efficacy. Because they have been less exposed to influenza viruses, children < 9 years old need two doses separated by 4 or more weeks when vaccinated against influenza for the first time.[12]

Vaccine efficacy varies with the degree of matching to circulating viruses. Efficacy also varies with the recipient's immune competence (eg, age, underlying illness). Influenza vaccine is about 90% effective in preventing illness in healthy young adults and reduces illness by about 30% to 40% among frail elderly patients. Despite this reduction in illness prevention, older vaccinees are still two to four times less likely to be hospitalized, develop pneumonia or die than their associates who decline influenza vaccine.

Influenza vaccine is recommended for several high-risk groups:

- Everyone ≥ 65 years old, even if perfectly healthy.
- People ≥ 6 months old with chronic illness (eg, residents of long-term care facilities, people 6 months to 18 years old on aspirin chronically). See the table titled "Diseases and Medications Indicating Need for Influenza and Pneumococcal Vaccine".
- Barrier groups that might otherwise infect high-risk people: Health-care providers, home-care workers, employees of long-term care facilities, household members of high-risk people.
- Others: Pregnant women (because of an increased rate of complications if infected), essential community workers (eg, police, fire, ambulance), international travelers, those living in crowded circumstances (eg, dormitories), anyone who wishes to lower the likelihood of influenza.

Influenza vaccine <u>cannot</u> cause influenza. The viruses are completely killed by formaldehyde during manufacture. Some people are incubating an influenza, rhinovirus or adenovirus infection at the time of vaccination, which may lead to a coincidental runny nose during the week after vaccination. This coincidence cannot be avoided. Do not blame the vaccine.

Pneumococcal Disease

Pneumococcal disease is caused by *Streptococcus pneumoniae,* a gram-positive bacillus. This disease group causes some 40,000 deaths each year, making it the leading cause of vaccine-preventable death in the US. Antibiotic-resistant strains of *S. pneumoniae* are becoming more common, up to 30% of isolates in some areas. These infections lead to more than 400,000 hospitalizations year after year.[13-16]

Pneumococcal disease has three major manifestations: Pneumonia, bacteremia and meningitis. Despite appropriate use of antibiotics, about 500,000 cases of pneumococcal pneumonia occur each year in this country with a 5% case-fatality ratio. Roughly ⅓ of community-acquired pneumonias and ½ of hospital-acquired lung infections are pneumococcal pneumonia. It is a common complication of infection with influenza or measles viruses. Pneumococcal bacteremia strikes 50,000 people per year, of whom 20% die despite antibiotic therapy. About 3000 cases of pneumococcal meningitis occur each year with a 30% case-fatality ratio despite antibiotics. The pneumococcal form represents 20% of all bacterial meningitis. Neurologic sequelae after this type of infection are common. Case-fatality ratios are higher among the elderly than among younger adults.

A polysaccharide capsule on pneumococcal bacteria confers virulence and is the basis for developing immunity. Pneumococcal vaccine consists of these purified polysaccharides. This vaccine reduces the likelihood of invasive disease by 60% to 70%. Efficacy falls with advancing age or underlying illness. Polysaccharide vaccines are not effective in children < 2.

The first pneumococcal vaccine, containing six polysaccharides, was developed by E. R. Squibb & Sons in 1947. Because prescribers preferred the new drug, penicillin, sales were insufficient for the product to be commercially viable. Thus, the Squibb vaccine was withdrawn in 1954.[3,12] A 14-valent vaccine was licensed in 1977. The current 23-valent vaccine followed in 1983. A 0.5 ml vaccine dose contains 25 mcg each of 23 polysaccharide types, accounting for 88% of bacteremic pneumococcal disease. These 23 antigens evoke antibodies that cross-react with pneumococcal types causing another 8% of the disease.

Most people need just a single dose of pneumococcal vaccine. One revaccination is recommended for recipients of the 14-valent vaccine at highest risk of fatal disease, (eg, people without spleens). One revaccination after a 5-year interval is recommended for recipients of the 23-valent vaccine at highest risk of fatal disease (eg, asplenia) or rapid decline in antibody levels (eg, nephrotic syndrome).[3,13] Also, patients with an immunosuppressive disorder or on immunosuppresive therapy. Give a second dose of this vaccine to people ≥ 65 years of age if they were < 65 years old when they received the first dose and if that dose was ≥ 5 years ago. Revaccinate children after 3 years if they would be ≤ 10 years old at revaccination.

Take Every Opportunity

Half to ⅔ of the people who die of influenza and pneumococcal disease were hospitalized in the 5 years preceding their death but were not vaccinated. Over 90% of these people visited a physician as an outpatient in the year preceding their death but were not vaccinated. Despite these contacts with the healthcare system, clinicians failed to capitalize on the chance to protect these people from deadly infection.[17-19]

Millions of people are vulnerable to death or debilitating disease from influenza or pneumococcal disease. Even in its milder forms, influenza causes many lost days of work and school each year. Influenza can cost the economy at least $12 billion during major epidemics.

Influenza and pneumococcal vaccines help elderly people living in the community stay healthy. In a 1994 study, influenza vaccination resulted in 46% less death, 48% to 57% fewer hospitalizations and net savings in direct medical costs of $117 per person vaccinated.[20] Mullooly, et al, found a 6:1 cost-savings ratio for influenza vaccine among the high-risk elderly in an HMO population.[21] In 1995, Nichol's group found that influenza vaccine reduces working adult health resource use by 25% fewer respiratory illnesses, 43% fewer days of sick leave, 44% fewer physician visits and net savings in direct medical costs of $46 per person vaccinated.[22]

Diseases & Medications Indicating Need for Influenza & Pneumococcal Vaccines[12]
(applies to both adults and children)

Disease	Medications
Heart disease (eg, congestive heart failure, myocardial infarction, heart anomalies)	Digoxin, warfarin, nitroglycerin, diuretics, others
Lung disease (eg, emphysema, COPD, asthma)	Albuterol, zafirlukast, ipratropium, theophylline, others
Metabolic (eg, diabetes)	Insulin, oral hypoglycemics, others
Healthy people ≥ 65 years	Any medication or none at all
Kidney disease (eg, renal dysfunction, nephrotic syndrome)	Allopurinol, azathioprine, others
Juvenile arthritis	Children on chronic aspirin therapy
HIV infection	Zidovudine, protease inhibitors, others
Hemophilia	Coagulation factors, others
Tuberculosis	Rifampin, pyrazinamide, others
Hemoglobinopathies (eg, sickle cell disease)	Hydroxyurea, others
Cancers (eg, Hodgkin's disease, lymphoma, multiple myeloma)	Alkylating agents, antimetabolites, interferons, mitotic inhibitors, others
Immunosuppression, various	IGIV, cyclosporine, others

Hepatitis B

Even though effective vaccines have been available since 1981, hepatitis B infection rates have fallen only slightly. Hepatitis B infection is still a major cause of disease in North America and even more so around the world. More than 300,000 yearly infections occurred in the US as recently as 1990, with 10,000 to 15,000 hospitalizations and 5000 deaths each year. Deaths can be broken down as follows: 400 caused by fulminant disease, 1500 caused by liver cancer and 4000 caused by cirrhosis.[1,4,9,14,23]

The rate fell to about 150,000 to 200,000 infections per year by 1995. Hepatitis B is the most common cause of chronic viremia on the globe with over 200 million carriers worldwide. Hepatitis B is a major cause of liver cancer, and only tobacco is a more common cause of cancer.

Hepatitis B infection has an incubation period of 6 weeks to 6 months. About 50% of infections are asymptomatic. Disease is characterized by jaundice, yellow skin, yellow eyes and dark urine. Acute cases involve fulminant hepatitis and hospitalization. Chronic infection results in cirrhosis, hepatocellular carcinoma and death. The primary route of transmission involves blood or body fluids. Subclinical infections are contagious for 1 to 2 months before and after onset.

The most common method of hepatitis B transmission is heterosexual contact (45%). About 15% of transmission is by homosexual contact, 12% by intravenous (IV) drug use, 3% is from household contact and 2% is among healthcare workers. About 25% of hepatitis B infections are not associated with any identifiable risk factor for transmission. The people most in danger include people exposed to blood products, certain immigrants, people in institutions for the developmentally disabled, contact with and partners of hepatitis B carriers, certain travelers, IV drug users, people with multiple sexual partners and some prison inmates.

Hepatitis B vaccines are highly effective in preventing infection, and reduce disease risk by about 80% to 95% after 3 doses. These inactivated viral vaccines consist of purified hepatitis B surface antigen (HBsAg) found on the outer viral coat. The purified antigen is immunogenic but not infectious. The first vaccine (*Heptavax-B* by Merck) was produced from human serum and available from 1981 to 1991.

More recently, recombinant HBsAg has been harvested from brewer's yeast. Merck's *Recombivax-HB* was licensed in 1986. SmithKline Beecham's *Engerix-B* was licensed in 1989. The two brands are prophylactically equivalent, but the volume and dose of antigen varies depending on age, package and brand. People started on one brand can use the other brand to complete their three-dose series after adjusting to the appropriate volume and dose of antigen for the brand used. Newborn children of HBsAg-positive mothers should receive hepatitis B vaccine and hepatitis B immune globulin (HBIG).[12]

The prevalence of infection increases with age as follows: 85% among adults, 8% among adolescents, 4% among children and 4% perinatal. Hepatitis B is the most common vaccine-preventable disease among children. Unfortunately, hepatitis B immunization of children lags behind that of other pediatric vaccines.

Although occupational health requirements have led healthcare workers to be highly vaccinated against this disease, only 10% to 20% of the highest risk adults are immunized against hepatitis B. Unfortunately, target ing healthcare workers and others at increased risk with vaccines is insufficient to stop the epidemic. Universal immunization of infants, children and adolescents, begun in 1991, is essential but not yet fully adopted. Targeted immunization of selected adults is still important. A pool of 1 to 1.25 million chronic carriers live in the US. The major risk factor in becoming a carrier is infection age. The odds are 90% at birth, 50% at 1 year of age and 10% after 5 years of age.[1,8,14,23-24]

All infants, adolescents and high-risk adults need protection from hepatitis B. Among adults, focus on people with multiple sexual partners or sexually transmitted diseases, IV drug users, dialysis patients, hemophiliacs, prisoners, immigrants and certain other subgroups.

"Childhood" Diseases

Americans can be very proud of their childhood immunization programs. Compulsory immunization laws result in immunization rates of 98% or higher among American children entering kindergarten or first grade. The rate of disease and death from polio, tetanus, diphtheria, pertussis, measles, mumps, rubella, *Haemophilus influenzae* type b (Hib) and other diseases have plummeted to a minuscule fraction of their former levels. These dangerous bacteria and viruses are still present in our environment. Only our ongoing commitment to immunization keeps American children and adults safe. For every $1 spent on these vaccines, an average of $10 is saved that would otherwise have been spent on managing the disease.

The successes discussed in the preceding paragraph correspond to 5- and 6-year-olds, unfortunately. Many of our preschool children suffer from major breaches in their immune protection. Twenty-five percent to 40% of preschoolers are unimmunized or underimmunized. In some communities, the fraction unprotected is > 60%. In Texas, before the "Shots Across Texas" program began, about 60% of 2-year-olds needed one or more vaccines to be completely immunized. At that time, over 4400 Texas children < 5 years of age developed measles; 14 of these children died.

Although childhood diseases have largely been conquered, they will come back to haunt us if we do not sustain high rates of immunity among children. These diseases include diphtheria, tetanus, pertussis, Hib, measles, mumps, rubella and poliomyelitis. We need to close the gap and deliver vaccines to these children if we are to reduce the > 5000 cases of pertussis, 3.5 million cases of chickenpox, 2000 cases of invasive Hib disease and several thousand cases each of measles, mumps and rubella. The high rates of hepatitis B among children and adolescents was discussed above. Tragically, each year we suffer roughly 25 deaths from pertussis, 50 to 100 deaths from chickenpox, 100 deaths from Hib disease, 50 deaths from measles, a dozen cases of congenital rubella syndrome and several hundred deaths from hepatitis B. Preventable infections will return to plague us if we do not maintain high vaccination rates.[2-4,14,24-26]

Measles

Measles is one of the most highly contagious of all infections. It is communicable from 4 days before to 4 days after rash appears, but measles is more than just a rash. Complications of measles include diarrhea (8%), otitis media (7%), pneumonia (6%, the most common cause of measles-induced death), encephalitis (0.1%) and death (0.2%). A resurgence in measles from 1989 to 1991 produced more than 55,000 cases and 200 deaths, most among unvaccinated preschool children. Another major cause was vaccine failure, caused by doses given too early, mishandled vaccine, mislabeled records or unresponsiveness.

Since 1991, the national policy has been to give two measles-mumps-rubella (MMR) vaccine doses. Two different recommendations for the timing of the second MMR dose have been proposed. The CDC's Advisory Committee on Immunization Practices (ACIP), considering the capabilities of the nation's health clinics, initially recommended the second dose between 4 and 6 years of age. This strategy takes advantage of the states' school-entry requirements. The American Academy of Pediatrics (AAP), recommended the second dose between 11 and 12 years of age. This approach lowers the vulnerable pool of children sooner. Since 1995, the ACIP and AAP have agreed to recommend either age, depending on individual circumstances. The most important issue is to focus on administering those second doses.

Adults born since 1957 need a second dose of MMR. Those most at risk include college students, healthcare workers and international travelers. There is no need to vaccinate against measles if the person is immune by serologic evidence, physician diagnosis or records of two vaccine doses. Even so, adult women may still need protection from rubella to protect their unborn children.

Mumps

Mumps virus, like the cause of measles, is a paramyxovirus. Inflammation of the parotid glands, parotitis, occurs in 30% to 40% of cases; 20% are fully asymptomatic. Mumps can be complicated by CNS involvement (15%, eg, aseptic meningitis), inflammation of the testes (orchitis, 20% to 50% in postpubertal males), permanent deafness (1 per 20,000) or death (1 to 3 per 10,000).

Mumps vaccine is a live, attenuated viral vaccine first licensed in 1968. It reduces disease risk by 95%. Immunize all infants > 12 months old, as well as susceptible adolescents and adults without documented immunity.

Rubella

Rubella is caused by a togavirus and is typically a mild disease. The connection between maternal infection and infant cataracts and heart defects was first recognized in 1941. This devastating condition came to be called congenital rubella syndrome (CRS), and also can involve deafness, microcephaly, mental retardation, bone alterations, miscarriage and liver and spleen damage. A worldwide pandemic of rubella occurred in 1963 to 1964, with 20,000 CRS cases in the US.

Lymphadenopathy develops in the second week with a rash developing 14 to 17 days after exposure. Half the cases may be asymptomatic. Arthralgia or arthritis develops after infection, rarely among children, and affects 50% to 70% of adult women who contract rubella. Thrombocytopenia purpura occurs in one in 3000 cases, and encephalitis in one in 5000. The public-health importance of rubella immunization is in avoiding CRS.

Live, attenuated rubella virus vaccines were first licensed in 1969 and improved in 1979. They are about 95% effective. Immunize all infants > 12 months old, as well as susceptible adolescents and adults without documented immunity. Physician or personal history of disease is not considered reliable.

Because of the devastating nature of CRS, there is great reluctance to give the live, albeit attenuated, vaccine to pregnant women. To appropriately screen a woman of child-bearing age, ask if she is pregnant or likely to become pregnant in the next 3 months. Explain the theoretical need to avoid pregnancy, and do not vaccinate those who say yes. Nonetheless, inadvertent pregnancies may occur among vaccine recipients. Of 324 live births monitored by the CDC among women who were vaccinated while pregnant or shortly before becoming pregnant, zero cases of CRS were observed. This standard for pregnancy screening has been used for more than two decades and no risk from vaccination in fertile women is evident.

Varicella

Varicella-zoster virus is a herpes virus that causes two forms of disease. The primary infection is varicella or chickenpox; three to four million cases occur each year in the US. After these cases resolve clinically, the virus remains dormant in nerve cells. When dormant viruses reactivate, the condition is known as herpes zoster, often called shingles. Postherpetic neuralgia from shingles can persist for a year.[25]

Varicella begins with a prodromal period, then pruritic vesicles develop, mostly on the trunk. Transmission is primarily respiratory, via airborne droplets, or direct contact with lesions 1 to 2 days before or 4 to 5 days after onset of rash. Roughly 87% of those who are susceptible to chickenpox and are exposed to it will develop the disease.

Varicella is more than just a rash. Its complications can include secondary bacterial infection of lesions with group A streptococci that is difficult to treat. Other complications might involve cerebellar ataxia, encephalitis or pneumonia. Three of every 1000 chickenpox cases are hospitalized each year, roughly 9000 times per year in the US. Death occurs in 1 of every 60,000 cases of varicella, roughly 50 to 100 deaths per year. Varicella is most risky when it infects healthy adults, immunocompromised people and newborns whose mothers developed the chickenpox rash 5 days before to 48 hours after delivery. Healthy adults have a case-fatality ratio 25 times higher than that of healthy children.

About 15% of people who get chickenpox will develop zoster at some point. Zoster is most often linked with aging, immunosuppression, intrauterine exposure or contracting varicella before reaching 18 months of age. Patients with zoster can transmit the virus to those susceptible to varicella.

Varicella vaccine was first developed in Japan in 1974 and then subjected to extensive testing. The current vaccine was licensed in the US in March

1995. It is a live, attenuated virus vaccine that reduces the risk of disease by 95%. Even in the few cases where disease among vaccine recipients does occur, it is far milder, often with < 10 lesions rather than the 200 or more lesions expected. Our national policy is to immunize all susceptible children 12 to 18 months of age, as well as the 5% to 15% of adolescents and adults who are susceptible. An oral history of this disease is considered reliable because chickenpox is so unique. Adolescents and adults need two doses of vaccine, rather than the single dose given to children.[12,25]

Diphtheria

Diphtheria is caused by *Corynebacterium diphtheriae,* a gram-positive, toxigenic bacillus. This disease can involve any mucous membrane: Most often, an exudative pharyngitis develops, forming a pseudo-membrane that may extend into the airway. Complications result from the bacteria's toxin, including myocarditis, neuritis and death. A 10% case-fatality ratio is common, although the risk of death is higher in children and the elderly.

Diphtheria was the leading cause of all deaths in the early 1900s, primarily striking children. Now it is rarely seen in the US, but diphtheria bacteria still circulate. Most cases now occur among adults; 20% to 60% of American adults are susceptible. An epidemic of diphtheria in Russia, Ukraine and nearby republics reminds us of the need to sustain diphtheria immunity among our population.

Immunity is conferred by immunizing with diphtheria toxoid produced by inactivating the bacterial toxin with formaldehyde. Diphtheria toxoid is one of the key ingredients in diphtheria-tetanus-pertussis (DTP) vaccine, diphtheria-tetanus toxoids for children (DT) and tetanus-diphtheria toxoids for adults (Td). The adult form contains ⅓ the dose of diphtheria toxoid included in pediatric vaccines to avoid local reactions.

Diphtheria toxoid is estimated to be about 95% effective. Standard procedures call for four or five doses of DTP as a child followed by Td doses every 10 years.

Tetanus

Tetanus is caused by *Clostridium tetani,* an anaerobic gram-positive bacillus. Tetanus spores are everywhere, found in soil, dust and feces. Tetanus toxin binds in the CNS, blocking neurotransmitters and preventing muscle relaxation. The disease is characterized by trismus (lockjaw), difficulty swallowing (or suckling), muscle rigidity and spasms (persisting 3 to 4 weeks) and death. The case-fatality ratio for tetanus is 30% higher among the elderly. Other complications can include bone fractures, pneumonia and strangulation.

About 50 to 100 cases of tetanus are reported each year in the US, primarily among the elderly. This level of disease is probably an underestimate of the true rate. Tetanus is not just a "rusty nail" disease. In the US, 40% of tetanus cases are associated with puncture wounds, with other cases associated with lacerations, abrasions, chronic wounds, IV drug use or diabetes. Ten percent are from unknown causes, perhaps undetected punctures. In one survey, ⅓ of tetanus cases came from an indoor injury.

Patients labeled as "allergic to tetanus shots" may actually have had serum sickness to tetanus antitoxin produced from equine serum. This antitoxin was replaced in the late 1950s by tetanus immune globulin from human plasma. Immediate-hypersensitivity reactions, such as anaphylaxis, can be a contraindication to future doses of tetanus toxoid. Getting serum sickness from antitoxic serum is irrelevant when deciding whether to give tetanus toxoid. Careful history reporting may clarify the issue.

Like its diphtheria counterpart, tetanus toxoid is produced by treating tetanus toxin with formaldehyde. Do not stock plain tetanus toxoid to immunize adults. Instead, use tetanus-diphtheria toxoids (Td), to sustain people's immunity. Efficacy is essentially 100% for this drug. The standard schedule includes four or five doses of DTP as a child followed by Td doses every 10 years.

Everyone needs protection against tetanus. Most cases of tetanus occur among adults; 40% to 85% of American adults are susceptible. Older women are more likely to be at risk than men because fewer of them were vaccinated during Armed Forces service during World War II.

Pertussis

Pertussis, or whooping cough, is caused by *Bordetella pertussis,* a gram-negative bacillus. The disease begins with a catarrhal stage with 1 to 2 weeks of a normal cough and slight fever. Next comes a paroxysmal ("whooping") cough of 1 to 6 weeks duration. The characteristic "whoop" or gasp results from inspiratory effort against a closed glottis. Convalescence from pertussis can take months.

Pertussis is extremely contagious. The disease can be complicated by pneumonia (9% of cases), seizures, encephalopathy and hypoxia. About 34% of cases are hospitalized. The worst cases of disease occur among children < 5 years old. This is troublesome because half the current cases occur among those < 1 year old. Two of every 1000 children who develop the disease die. These data highlight the importance of vaccinating young children on schedule. Experts at CDC describe it as unfair to deny pertussis vaccine to children with underlying neurologic conditions, such as seizure disorders, stable epilepsy, cerebral palsy or a ventricular shunt. Do postpone immunization with pertussis vaccine until after evolving neurologic conditions resolve.

The original pertussis vaccines are called whole-cell vaccines (or DTwP). This refers to including all bacterial components in the vaccine formula after inactivation with formaldehyde. The standard schedule includes five doses. Its efficacy is 70% to 90%, with protection persisting 5 to 10 years. From ⅓ to ½ of the children who get this vaccine develop redness, swelling or pain at the injection site. Fever > 105°F develops in three per 1000 recipients with hypotonic episodes in one per 1750 and (usually febrile) convulsions in one per 1750. Much public debate has occurred over whether pertussis vaccine leads to encephalopathy. Immunization with pertussis vaccine may be associated with acute encephalopathy, perhaps at a rate of one per 100,000 to one million recipients but without any lasting problems. There seems to be no causal association between pertussis vaccine and chronic neurologic damage. The ACIP and AAP empirically suggest giving acetaminophen every 4 hours for 24 hours after receiving DTwP to decrease the risk of a febrile convulsion.

If a child develops either a serious allergic reaction or encephalopathy within 7 days after DTP immunization, he or she should not receive any further doses of pertussis vaccine but rather DT. The following events after DTwP administration also serve as contraindications to future doses of DTwP unless there is a pertussis outbreak in the community: Temperature > 105°F, collapse or shock-like state, persistent inconsolable crying > 3 hours or convulsions with or without fever. None of these events has been associated with permanent brain injury.

More recently, so-called acellular pertussis vaccines (or DTaP) have been developed that contain just some specific components of pertussis bacteria. These components include pertussis toxin, filamentous hemagglutinin, agglutinogen and pertactin. Four or five doses of DTaP form the standard regimen for children. Acellular pertussis vaccines have the advantage of causing fewer injection-site reactions and less fever, irritability, drowsiness and high-pitched crying. DTaP is steadily superseding DTwP as the preferred vaccine.

Experts agree that adolescents and adults are a major reservoir of pertussis bacteria in the community and a source of children infections. Acellular pertussis vaccines may eventually be appropriate for older ages.

Poliomyelitis

Poliomyelitis is caused by three types of poliovirus. Poliovirus enters the body through the mouth, then replicates in the nasopharynx and GI tract. It enters the CNS via the bloodstream. Some 95% of infections are asymptomatic but contagious.[26]

Minor non-CNS illness occurs in 2% to 5% of polio infections with nonparalytic aseptic meningitis in another 1% to 2%. Paralytic disease occurs in 1 in 200 to 1000 infections. Anterior horn cells of the spinal cord are most frequently damaged, leaving sensory function intact but impairing motor function. Thus, each observed case of poliomyelitis implies several hundred inapparent infections.

Polio was a major source of fear among the population in the 1950s. The public rejoiced at the success of Salk's inactivated poliovirus vaccine (IPV) in 1955. Sabin's live, attenuated oral poliovirus vaccine (OPV) was licensed in 1963. Disease rates fell rapidly after widespread vaccine distribution began, which was 95% to 99% effective in preventing disease.

OPV has the advantages of inducing GI mucosal immunity, providing long-lasting protection, being easy to administer and spreading to susceptible contacts. This last advantage is actually a double-edged sword. Extraordinarily rare, about 1 in every 2.6 million OPV doses distributed can revert to virulence from their attenuated form. This amounts to 5 to 10 cases of vaccine-associated paralytic poliomyelitis (VAPP) per year. In such cases, OPV can cause paralytic poliomyelitis instead of preventing it. VAPP is far more likely among immunocompromised people than healthy people. The risk is also somewhat elevated for first doses compared with later doses.

IPV, on the other hand, has no known risks. Because it is inactivated, it can never cause poliomyelitis. Unfortunately, it does not induce GI mucosal immunity. IPV is the only appropriate vaccine for immunocompromised children and household contacts of people with immunodeficiency.

To achieve the best mix of the advantages of IPV and OPV, our national policy for immunizing infants against poliovirus changed in January 1997 to a sequential schedule of two IPV doses followed by two OPV doses. Alternate acceptable regimens include four doses of OPV or four doses of IPV. If a household member has never been vaccinated against polio, vaccinate the infant. Then remind the family to be especially careful to wash their hands after changing diapers. Consider immunizing that household member. Give adults a booster IPV dose before travel overseas.

Poliomyelitis was endemic in the US from about 1843 to 1979. Most people were infected as children. As sanitation improved, the age at onset of infection was delayed to later in life when infection is more risky. The Western hemisphere has been disease-free for several years although there is still a risk of introducing disease by international travelers from Africa or Asia. The world's goal is to eradicate poliovirus from the planet by the year 2000.

Haemophilus influenzae type b

Haemophilus influenzae type b (Hib) is an aerobic, gram-negative bacillus. Like the pneumococcus, the Hib polysaccharide capsule is responsible for virulence and immunity. Until recently, Hib was the leading cause of bacterial meningitis among children < 5 years of age, striking one of every 200 children. Two-thirds of these cases occurred among children < 18 months of age.

Hib invasive disease involves meningitis (50% to 65% of infections), epiglottitis (15% to 20%), pneumonia, osteomyelitis, arthritis, cellulitis or bacteremia. It is spread by respiratory transmission from asymptomatic carriers. Before Hib vaccine was widely used, 5% to 15% of children were colonized with Hib at any given time. This led to 20,000 invasive cases and 1000 deaths per year in the US.

Hib invasive disease can be complicated by deafness with neurologic sequelae in 15% to 30% of survivors. Hib was the leading cause of acquired mental retardation. It had a case-fatality ratio of 2% to 5% despite antibiotics.

Groups to be vaccinated against Hib include all infants, plus anyone without a spleen or with sickle-cell disease, Hodgkin's disease, hematologic neoplasms, immunosuppression or HIV infection.

Purified Hib polysaccharide vaccines were first licensed in 1985, but they were not effective in children < 12 months old. The first protein-conjugated Hib vaccines, introduced in 1987, were effective in infants as young as 6 weeks of age. The protein carriers to which the Hib polysaccharides are conjugated make the Hib antigens T-cell dependent, improving antibody activity and booster responses. Three conjugated Hib vaccines are available for infant use. The dosing schedules vary slightly, depending on brand. The brands are generally interchangeable, if needed.

Widespread use of Hib vaccines lowered the number of disease cases from 20,000 in 1985 to 259 in 1995. Without Hib invasive disease, fewer sick children are hospitalized. Children < 24 months old who develop invasive Hib disease do not develop immunity and should still be immunized.

"Childhood" Disease Among Adolescents and Adults

"Childhood" diseases do not limit themselves to children. These statistics on vaccine-preventable diseases show the importance of vaccinating adolescents and adults at every opportunity.[1-5,9-10,12,14,25-27]

Hepatitis B: In the US, most people acquire hepatitis B virus (HBV) infection as adolescents or young adults. In 1994 an estimated 140,000 people, primarily young adults, were infected with HBV.

Measles: Between 1990 and 1994, 47% of reported cases of measles occurred in people ≥ 20 years of age, compared with only 10% from 1960 to 1964 (CDC unpublished data).

Tetanus: The prevalence of immunity decreases during the early teen years, leaving 15% to 36% unprotected (CDC unpublished data).

Diphtheria: Surveys conducted since 1977 indicate that 22% to 62% of adults 18 to 39 years of age may lack protective levels of circulating antitoxin against diphtheria.

Varicella: By age 11 to 12 years, over 20% of adolescents have not developed chickenpox and remain susceptible to varicella (CDC unpublished data). The rate of complications, including death, is much higher in people who develop chickenpox when they are ≥ 15 years of age.

Influenza: Over eight million children in the US have at least one high-risk condition warranting annual influenza vaccination.

Pneumococcal disease: About 340,000 people in the US 2 to 18 years of age have chronic illnesses associated with increased risk of pneumococcal disease. Several million more have asthma and should be immunized.

Hepatitis A virus infection: The highest rates of disease occur among people 5 to 14 years of age (CDC unpublished data).

Identify Those in Need of Vaccination

The people needing influenza and pneumococcal vaccines include:

- Adults and children with chronic pulmonary or cardiovascular disorders, including children with asthma.
- Adults and children who need regular medical follow-up or have had hospitalization during the previous year for chronic metabolic diseases (including diabetes mellitus), renal dysfunction, problems

related to hemoglobin or any form of immunosuppression (including that caused by medications).
- Residents of nursing homes and other chronic-care facilities housing people of any age with chronic medical conditions; many of them also need pneumococcal vaccine.
- Children and teenagers (6 months to 18 years of age) who receive long-term aspirin therapy and, therefore, may be at risk of developing Reye's syndrome if they contract influenza.
- Age ≥ 65 years, even if otherwise healthy. People in this age group account for 80% of influenza deaths.

A survey of Minnesota nursing homes showed that the influenza vaccination rate was 84%, but 35% of homes failed to offer vaccine to residents newly admitted during the influenza immunization season.[28] Sixty-nine percent of homes had written policies for influenza vaccination, ⅓ had policies for pneumococcal vaccine and only 16% for tetanus-diphtheria (Td). Twelve-month immunization rates were 12% and 3% for these latter two vaccines, respectively. With low baseline immunity rates, these rates probably leave much of this population vulnerable. Influenza vaccination of employees averaged 33%. Few sites evaluated immunization practices in their quality-assurance programs.

All children need to have an immune armor inventory, especially preschool children. Remind parents of the importance of on-time immunization to protect their children while they are toddlers.

Detailed information about people without spleens or with various forms of immunodeficiency is presented in chapter five, "Special Situations." Issues related to pregnant or lactating women and other situations are considered, as well.

Members of some minority groups are less likely to have been immunized than the rest of the population. For example, serious discrepancies exist between African-Americans and European-Americans, as well as between Hispanics and non-Hispanics. Immunization rates for African-American and European-American women ≥ 65 years of age for influenza vaccine were 29% and 54%, for pneumococcal vaccine, 14% and 29% and for tetanus toxoid, 22% and 28%. For senior Hispanic women, the three rates were 38%, 14% and 25%. Among adults with diabetes mellitus, influenza vaccination rates were 13% and 37% for African-Americans and European-Americans, respectively. Racial variations are accounted for, in part, by differences in factors such as maternal education, maternal age, socioeconomic status and family size.

References

[1] National Vaccine Advisory Committee. *Adult Immunization.* Washington, DC: Government Printing Office, 1994.

[2] Advisory Committee on Immunization Practices. General recommendations on immunization. *MMWR* 1994;43(RR-1):1-38.

[3] Peter G, ed. 1994 *Red Book: Report of the Committee on Infectious Diseases,* 23rd ed. Elk Grove Village, IL: American Academy of Pediatrics, 1994.

[4] Hinman AR, Orenstein WA. Public health considerations. In: Plotkin SA, Mortimer EA Jr., ed. *Vaccines,* 2nd ed. Philadelphia: WB Saunders, 1994:903-32.

[5] Centers for Disease Control & Prevention. Quarterly immunization table. *MMWR* 1997;46:88.

[6] Centers for Disease Control & Prevention. Influenza and pneumococcal vaccination coverage levels among persons aged ≥ 65 years – United States, 1973-1993. *MMWR* 1995;44:506-7,513-5.

[7] Centers for Disease Control & Prevention. Pneumonia and influenza death rates – United States, 1979-1994. *MMWR* 1995;44:535-7.

[8] Centers for Disease Control & Prevention. Mortality patterns – US, 1993. *MMWR* 1996;45:161-4.

[9] Advisory Committee on Immunization Practices. Update on adult immunization: Recommendations of the Immunization Practices Advisory Committee. *MMWR* 1991;40(RR-12):1-94.

[10] Gardner P, Schaffner W. Immunization of adults. *N Engl J Med* 1993;328:1252-8.

[11] Advisory Committee on Immunization Practices. Prevention and control of influenza: Recommendations of the Immunization Practices Advisory Committee. *MMWR* 1997;46(RR-9):1-25.

[12] Grabenstein JD. *ImmunoFacts: Vaccines & Immunologic Drugs.* St. Louis: Facts and Comparisons, May 1997.

[13] Advisory Committee on Immunization Practices. Prevention of pneumococcal disease. *MMWR* 1997;46(RR-8):1-24.

[14] American College of Physicians. *Guide for Adult Immunization,* 3rd ed. Philadelphia: American College of Physicians, 1994.

[15] McBean AM, Babish JD, Prihoda R. The utilization of pneumococcal polysaccharide vaccine among elderly Medicare beneficiaries, 1985 through 1988. *Arch Intern Med* 1991;151:2009-16.

[16] Butler JC, Hofmann J, Cetron MS, et al. The continued emergence of drug-resistant *Streptococcus pneumoniae* in the United States: An update from the Centers for Disease Control & Prevention's Pneumococcal Sentinel Surveillance System. *J Infect Dis* 1996;174:986-93.

[17] Magnussen CR, Valenti WM, Mushlin AI. Pneumococcal vaccine strategies. *Arch Intern Med* 1984;144:1755-7.

[18] Fedson DS. Influenza and pneumococcal immunization strategies for physicians. *Chest* 1987;91:435-43.

[19] Williams WW, Hickson MA, Kane MA, et al. Immunization policies and vaccine coverage among adults: The risk for missed opportunities. *Ann Intern Med* 1988;108:616-25.

[20] Nichol KL, Margolis KL, Wuorenma J, et al. The efficacy and cost-effectiveness of vaccination against influenza among elderly persons living in the community. *N Engl J Med* 1994;331:778-84.

[21] Mullooly JP, Bennett MD, Hornbrook MC, et al. Influenza vaccination programs for elderly persons: Cost-effectiveness in a health maintenance organization. *Ann Intern Med* 1994;121:947-52.

[22] Nichol KL, Lind A, Margolis KL, et al. The effectiveness of vaccination against influenza in healthy, working adults. *N Engl J Med* 1995;333:889-93.

[23] Centers for Disease Control & Prevention. Update: Recommendations to prevent hepatitis B virus transmission – United States. *MMWR* 1995;44:574-5.

[24] Centers for Disease Control & Prevention. Recommended childhood immunization schedule – United States, 1997. *MMWR* 1997;46:35-40.

[25] Advisory Committee on Immunization Practices. Prevention of varicella: Recommendations of the Advisory Committee on Immunization Practices. *MMWR* 1995;44(RR-11):1-36.

[26] Advisory Committee on Immunization Practices. Poliomyelitis prevention in the United States: Introduction of a sequential vaccination schedule of inactivated poliovirus vaccine followed by oral poliovirus vaccine: Recommendations of the Advisory Committee on Immunization Practices. *MMWR* 1997;46(RR-3):1-25. Errata 1997;46:183.

[27] Advisory Committee on Immunization Practices. Prevention of hepatitis A through active or passive immunization: Recommendations of the Advisory Committee on Immunization Practices. *MMWR* 1996;45(RR-15):1-30.

[28] Nichol KL, Grimm MB, Peterson DC. Immunizations in long-term care facilities: Policies and practice. *J Am Geriatr Soc* 1996;44:349-55.

[29] Potter J, Stott DJ, Roberts MA, et al. Influenza vaccination of health care workers in long-term-care hospitals reduces the mortality of elderly patients. *J Infect Dis* 1997;175:1-6.

Table I. Immunization Recommendations Based On Personal Factors

Immunologic Drug	Occupation: Health-care workers	Occupation: Day-care workers	Occupation: Essential workers (police, fire, etc.)	Occupation: Animal & Lab workers	Occupation: Military personnel	Health Status: HIV-infected persons	Health Status: Other immuno-deficiencies	Health Status: Pregnant women[P]	Health Status: Persons with chronic illness[C]	Lifestyle & Other Factors: Travelers & Immigrants	Lifestyle & Other Factors: Nursing home & Institutional residents or staff	Lifestyle & Other Factors: Ethnic & Social groups	Lifestyle & Other Factors: Other groups
Routine													
Diphtheria & Tetanus	Td	Td	Td	Td	Td	Td	Td	Td	Td	Td	Td	Td	Td
Measles	+	+			+	HC	0	0		T,I		H	
Mumps	+	+			+	HC	0	0		T,I		H	
Rubella	+	+			+	HC	0	0,RT		T,I		H	
Haemophilus influenzae type b						+	AS	NC	S	I		H	
Hepatitis B	BX		BX	L (BX)	BX,T	+	HD	HP	HD	T,I	BX,MR,PI	AP,H,LS	BX,CC,PE
Influenza A & B	+	+	+		+	+	+	NC	+	T,I	+	H	CS
Pneumococcal						+	+	NC	+	SR	SR	H	
Poliovirus[PV]	IPV	IPV		L	OPV	IPV	IPV	PP		T,I		H	CS
Unusual													
Adenovirus				L	BT	0	0	0					
Anthrax				A,L				RB					
Cholera				L	T			RB		T			
Hepatitis A	SR	SR		L	T	S	S	NC		T,I	SR	H,SR	PE,SR
Japanese encephalitis				L						T			
Meningococcal				L	BT,T	NC	AS	NC		T			
Plague				A,L	T			RB		T			
Rabies				A,L	T			NC		T			PE
Smallpox				L	BT	0	0	0	0				
Typhoid				lL	T	SQ	SQ	SQ,RB		T			CC
Varicella	SV	SV			SV	0	SV	0		T,I		H	
Yellow fever				L	T	0	0	RB		T			
BCG						0	0	0				B,H	
Tuberculin skin test	TST				TST	TST	SR	NC	SR	T,I	TST	H,SR	ADU CC

Key for Table I

\+ – Immunity needed. Vaccine indicated if patient is susceptible. Prescriber must still consider possible contraindications, as well as vaccination history.

O – Vaccine generally contraindicated. Certain isolated individuals may benefit from this vaccine. Consult detailed references.

A – Animal workers, including veterinarians and their assistants.

ADU – Alcoholics, IV drug abusers and medically under-served low-income populations.

AP – Alaskan natives, Pacific Islanders, immigrants and refugees from hepatitis B endemic ares (particularly Haiti, Africa and eastern Asia).

AS – Asplenic patients.

BT – Military recruits at basic training.

BX – If exposed to blood or other contaminated body fluids.

C – Chronic illnesses include: Hemodynamically significant cardiovascular disease, pulmonmary disease (eg, asthma, active tuberculosis, myasthenia gravis, cystic fibrosis, chronic obstructive pulmonary disease), diabetes mellitus, renal or hepatic dysfunction, sickle-cell and chronic hemolytic anemia, chronic alcoholism or cirrhosis and others.

CC – Close contacts of pathogen carriers or close contacts of infectious cases.

CS – Close contacts of susceptible patients.

H – When assessing the homeless, review status for all routine vaccines.

HC – HIV-infected children.

HD – Haemophilia, thalassemia, dialysis and renal failure patients.

HIV – Human immunodeficiency virus.

HP – Screen all pregnant women for HBsAg; vaccinate newborn infants of HBsAg+ mothers.

I – Selected immigrants based on origin, age and health; includes refugees, guest workers, foreign students and internationally adopted children.

IPV – Enhanced-potency inactive poliovirus vaccine (e-IPV).

L – Laboratory workers potentially exposed to the corresponding pathogen.

LS – Homosexual and bisexual men, intravenous drug abusers, prostitutes, heterosexually active persons with multiple sexual partners or recently acquired sexually transmitted disease.

MR – Clients and staff of institutions for the mentally or developmentally retarded.

NC – Not contraindicated.

OPV – Oral, attenuated poliovirus vaccine.

P – Includes women planning to become pregnant within 3 months.

PE – Used for post-exposure to prophylaxis.

PI – Prison inmates.

PP – Vaccinate pregnant women only if at high risk of exposure to poliovirus. OPV is acceptable if immediate protection is needed. Alternately, 2 doses of e-IPV may be used. Use e-IPV for women who previously received a complete primary series.

PV – When choosing between e-IPV and OPV, consult detailed references.

RB – Consider the risk-benefit ratio; vaccinate only if clearly needed.

RT – Screen all pregnant women for rubella antibody titer. If vaccine is needed, administer after delivery but before patient's discharge. Rh_o(D) immune globulin does not interfere with rubella vaccine.

S – Vaccine indicated for selected individuals in this category. See diagnosis and drug tables elsewhere in this book.

SC – Live, oral typhoid-vaccine capsules are contraindicated. Inactivated, subcutaneous vaccine may be acceptable. Consider risk-benefit ratio.

SR – Many in this category warrant vaccination, based on other risk ractors. See diagnosis and drug tables on the following pages.

SV – Women of childbearing potential if seronegative for varicella.

T – Selected travelers, depending on destinations and itinereary. For further information, telephone CDC's health requirements and recommendations 24-hour hotline: 404-332-4559.

Td – Adult-strength tetanus-diphtheria toxoids (Td) indicated at 10-year intervals. Wound-management guidelines are cited elsewhere.

TST – Many in this category warrant testing.

Diseases & Diagnoses Warranting Immunization

Disease/Diagnosis	Vaccine(s) Indicated
Age > 64 years, even if healthy	Influenza, pneumonia
Alcoholism, chronic	Pneumonia
Antibiotic allergies, multiple (especially penicillin and erythromycin)	Influenza, pneumonia
Anemia (chronic, severe) including sickle-cell and chronic hemolytic	Influenza, pneumonia
Artificial heart valve	Influenza, pneumonia
Aspirin therapy, long-term, in children	Influenza
Asplenia	Influenza, pneumonia
Asthma	Influenza, pneumonia
Atherosclerosis	Influenza, pneumonia
Azotemia	Influenza
Bedridden, chronically	Influenza, pneumonia
Cancer	Influenza, pneumonia
Cardiovascular disease ("altered circulatory dynamics")	Influenza, pneumonia
Cerebrospinal fluid leaks	Pneumonia
Cirrhosis	Pneumonia
Claudication, intermittent	Influenza, pneumonia
Congestive heart failure	Influenza, pneumonia
Cystic fibrosis	Influenza, pneumonia
Diabetes mellitus	Influenza, pneumonia
Dialysis, kidney	Influenza, hepatitis B, pneumonia
Hemophilia	Hepatitis B, hepatitis A
Hepatitis B, chronic carriers of	Hepatitis A
HIV infection	Influenza, pneumonia
Immunodeficiency, natural or induced	Influenza, pneumonia
Kidney disease, chronic	Influenza, pneumonia
Liver failure	Influenza, hepatitis A
Mitral stenosis	Influenza, pneumonia
Myasthenia gravis	Influenza, pneumonia
Nephrotic syndrome	Influenza, pneumonia
Panacinar emphysema (with use of $alpha_1$-protease inhibitor)	Hepatitis B
Pulmonary disease	Influenza, pneumonia
Renal failure	Influenza, pneumonia
Septral defect	Influenza, pneumonia
Sexually transmitted diseases, repeated	Hepatitis B, hepatitis A
Splenic dysfunction, asplenia	Influenza, pneumonia
Thalassemia	Hepatitis B
Transplantation, organ	Influenza, pneumonia
Tuberculosis, active	Influenza, pneumonia

Drugs Indicative of Diseases Warranting Immunization		
Category Title	Representative Drugs	Immunization-Indicating Disease States
ANTI-INFECTIVE DRUGS		
Antifungal antibiotics	Ketoconazole	Hyperadrenocorticism
Anti-influenza agents	Amantadine	Influenza A prophylaxis
Antimalarial agents	Chloroquine, hydroxychloroquine	Rheumatoid arthritis, travel to hepatitis-B endemic area
Antitubercular agents	Rifampin, pyrazinamide	Tuberculosis treatment
Antivirals	Zidovudine, didanosine	HIV infection
Sulfonamides	Sulfasalazine	Crohn's disease
ANTINEOPLASTIC DRUGS		
Alkylating agents	Cyclophosphamide	Cancer, various
Antimetabolites	Azathioprine	Glumerulonephritis, immunosuppression, nephrotic syndrome, cirrhosis
Interferons	Interferon-alfa	Cancer, hepatitis, various
Mitotic inhibitors	Etoposide	Cancer, various
BLOOD MODIFIERS		
Anticoagulants	Heparin, warfarin	Cardiovascular disease
Folic acid products	Leucovorin	Antagonist rescue, anemia
Hemorheologic agents	Pentoxifylline	Cardiovascular disease
Hemostatics	Coagulation factors VIII, IX	Hemophilia
Thrombolytic agents	Alteplase, streptokinase	Cardiovascular disease
CARDIOVASCULAR DRUGS		
Cardiac drugs	Digoxin, disopyramide	Cardiovascular disease
Diuretics	Furosemide	Congestive heart failure
Vasodilating agents	Dipyridamole, isosorbide nitroglycerin	Cardiovascular disease
CNS DRUGS		
Gold compounds	Auranofin	Rheumatoid arthritis
Heavy metal antagonists	Penicillamine	Rheumatoid arthritis
GI DRUGS		
Digestants	Pancreatin, pancrelipase	Cystic fibrosis
Miscellaneous GI drugs	Mesalamine	Crohn's disease
	Colchicine	Cirrhosis

Drugs Indicative of Diseases Warranting Immunization

Category Title	Representative Drugs	Immunization-Indicating Disease States
HORMONES		
Adrenal hormones	Corticosteroids	Asthma, certain anemias, immunosuppression
Adrenal steroid inhibitors	Aminoglutethimide, Trilostane	Hyperadrenocorticlism
Insulins	Insulins	Diabetes mellitus
Sulfonylureas	Glyburide	Diabetes mellitus
IMMUNOLOGIC DRUGS		
Immune globulins	IV immune globulin	Immunodeficiency
	Anti-thymocyte globulin	Organ transplant
	Muromonab-CD3	Organ transplant
Immunosuppressants	Cyclosporine	Organ transplant
RADIOISOTOPES		
Therapeutic isotopes	NaI-131, NaP-32	Certain cancers
RENAL DRUGS		
Agents for gout	Allopurinol	Renal calculi
Ammonia detoxicants	Potassium acid phosphate	Renal calculi
RESPIRATORY DRUGS		
Anticholinergic agents	Ipratropium	Pulmonary disease
Leukotriene receptor antagonists	Zafirlukast	Asthma
Parasympathomimetics	Pyridostigmine bromide	Myasthenia gravis
Respiratory smooth muscle relaxants	Aminophylline, theophylline	Pulmonary disease
Sympathomimetic agents	Albuterol	Pulmonary disease
Enzyme replacements	Alpha$_1$-protease inhibitor	Congenital panacinar emphysema

CHAPTER 3

The Science of Vaccinology: How Vaccines and Antibodies Work

Until recently, most health-science students received little formal education in immunology. Even those who had a course in immunology probably learned more about immunologic theory than practical applications about immunologic drugs. This chapter will give the basics to understand how to protect health with vaccines.

The basic scientific aspects of immunization and immunity are readily understood using a compare-contrast method. This section describes the key features of applied immunology using common examples.

The marvel of the human body includes the complicated coagulation and prostaglandin process to stop bleeding and produce inflammation. The hematopoietic process is similarly complex. Like these examples, the interplay of cells, antibodies and mediators in an immune response is incredibly intricate. Yet we are slowly peeling the onion that is the immune system, revealing more interrelationships and understanding more of its intricacies.

Vaccines Are Drugs

The FDA divides itself into a Center for Drug Evaluation & Research (CDER) and a Center for Biologics Evaluation & Research (CBER). The term "biologics" arose to differentiate drugs derived from microbes, animals, blood or allergens from more traditional drugs. "Traditional drugs" meaning drugs with discrete chemical structures derived from plants or manufactured synthetically.[1]

Despite FDA's partition, biologics are drugs too. The classic definition of a drug is an agent intended to diagnose, cure, mitigate, treat or prevent disease. Vaccines and antibodies fit this definition as drugs.

Cellular vs Humoral Immunity

First, we explore the areas where the sciences of immunology and pharmacy overlap, emphasizing immunopharmacology, which is the study of the effects of immunologic drugs on living organisms.[2-5]

Mechanisms of immune responses can be differentiated into humoral and cell-mediated types. Humoral immunity involves antibodies; cell-mediated immunity involves macrophages, other antigen-presenting cells and T-lymphocytes. The pathology of these two types of immune response can be distinguished by their speed: Immediate (eg, within minutes) or delayed (eg, within 24 to 72 hours).

Consider the dichotomy between the mumps vaccine (*Mumpsvax,* Merck) and mumps skin test antigen (*MSTA,* Pasteur-Mérieux-Connaught). Both are antigens, both contain viral proteins, yet their effects are different.

Antigens in *MSTA* interact with T-lymphocytes to produce the characteristic delayed-type hypersensitivity response similar to tuberculin. Live viruses in mumps vaccine evoke specific circulating antimump antibodies that help defend the body. Tetanus toxoid is used in both these modes:

1.) Induction of antitoxin antibodies when used as a vaccine,
2.) Evocation of a delayed-hypersensitivity response when used intradermally as an anergy test reagent.[6-7]

Active vs Passive Immunity

Active immunity develops in a person in response to infection or after giving a vaccine or toxoid. Sufficient active immunity to protect the host may take several weeks or months to induce but is generally long-lasting.[5,7]

Passive immunity is temporary immunity provided in the form of preformed, donated antitoxins or antibodies (eg, immune globulins) from another living host (either human or animal). Passive immunity protects almost immediately but only persists with the biological half-life of IgG, measured in weeks.

Hepatitis B vaccine and hepatitis B immune globulin illustrate this dichotomy well. The vaccine actively induces someone to produce his or her own antibodies against the hepatitis B virus (HBV). That person also produces memory B-cells that permit an accelerated antibody response upon exposure to the whole virus. Giving HBIG is essentially the loan of someone else's antibodies. If an HBIG recipient has not developed any specific anti-HBV antibody-producing plasma cells, the loaned antibodies are eventually catabolized and not replaced. In this respect, the immunity provided is only temporary. In some cases of post-exposure prophylaxis, vaccine and HBIG are given. That way, the patient gets immediate, transient protection from the antibodies while the vaccine elicits long-lasting but delayed immunity.

In some cases, simultaneous administration of active and passive immunity may induce a drug-drug interaction that interferes with development of active immunity. For example, measles vaccine should be given at least 4 weeks before or 6 to 8 weeks after administration of any immune globulin or other blood product that might contain antimeasle antibodies. Hepatitis B vaccine and HBIG do not appear to interfere with each other.

If someone is bitten by a rabid animal, two drugs are given: Rabies immune globulin (RIG) and rabies vaccine. RIG promptly delivers someone else's antibodies to the patient to help neutralize the rabies virus. These antibodies provide prompt protection, but that protection only persists for a few weeks. Giving antibodies in this way is called passive immunization.

Because rabies is a disease that incubates slowly, persistent immunity is needed to protect the patient. A five-dose rabies vaccine series will protect for several years, ample time for post-exposure protection. Humans take a couple weeks to produce antibodies after being vaccinated. Causing people to make their own antibodies is called active immunization. In the case of our bitten patient, RIG and rabies vaccine are needed for full protection. The first provides prompt but temporary help, and the other gives delayed but persistent defense.

Primary vs Booster Responses

After an initial or primary immunization, IgM antibodies appear within about 4 days and peak about 4 days later. IgG antibodies appear after about 7 days and peak in 10 to 14 days. IgG concentrations decline slowly as the antibodies bind to antigen or are naturally catabolized.

After time passes and specific memory B-lymphocytes develop, a later immunization yields an immune response that is qualitatively and quantitatively different. The secondary or booster dose induces IgG that appears earlier, persists longer and reaches a higher level. IgM concentrations increase slightly, but IgG antibodies clearly predominate after booster immunizations.

In practice, several vaccine doses may be needed for a basic series to induce sufficient memory B cells. Later, less frequent booster doses are needed to maintain protective antibody concentrations. For diphtheria and tetanus toxoids, five doses are given as a basic series to induce adequate antitoxin concentrations. Booster doses are then needed only every 10 years to maintain adequate immunity.

Some vaccines are protective beginning shortly after a single dose, such as influenza, measles-mumps-rubella, yellow fever and other vaccines. Others require several doses to achieve protective concentrations of antibodies. Several doses are more likely to be required if the recipient is an infant (eg, DTP, poliovirus, *Haemophilus influenzae* type b), if protection is needed urgently (eg, rabies) or if the person has not had much natural exposure to the microbe (eg, influenza in children).

Disease vs Infection

Vaccines provide differing kinds of protection depending on the pathogenic characteristics of the microorganism. Toxoids prevent intoxication through antigen-antibody neutralization. Measles vaccination prevents infection by that virus. Pertussis and *Haemophilus influenzae* type b (Hib) vaccines prevent the manifestations of infection or reduce disease severity more than they prevent infection or colonization itself.

Antiviral immune globulins (eg, CMV-IGIV) attack invading microbes directly. Antitoxin antibodies (eg, tetanus immune globulin, antivenins) neutralize circulating toxins primarily, instead of toxins that have already fixed to nerve tissue.

Local vs Circulating Antibodies

The greatest advantage of oral poliovirus vaccine is its ability to induce large quantities of IgA antibodies in the gastric mucosa. These antibodies provide the strongest immune defense at the microorganism's portal of entry into the human body. IPV and OPV induce protective concentrations of antipoliovirus IgG that circulates in the blood stream.[8]

Scientists are investigating intranasal administration of influenza vaccine and oral administration of cholera vaccine. These routes may improve immune defenses at a microbe's portal of entry, taking advantage of secretory immunity. This approach is already used for some veterinary vaccines.

Killed vs Live Vaccines

Killed or inactivated vaccines are composed of whole, killed microbes or certain microbial parts. These nonreplicating immunogens induce active immunity. Live, attenuated vaccines contain altered, weakened or avirulent microorganisms (either bacteria or viruses) and also induce active immunity. Live vaccines can be dangerous in an immunocompromised person who cannot mount an effective defense against even avirulent microbes. Attenuated vaccines are often more immunogenic than inactive vaccines and may induce serum antibody protection of longer duration. For example, a single dose of live yellow-fever vaccine induces immunity for 10 years while Japanese-encephalitis vaccine requires a three-dose series that persists for an uncertain period of time.

Consider the dichotomy between the injectable inactivated poliovirus vaccine (IPV) and oral poliovirus vaccine (OPV). The best known contrast among vaccines is that between the Salk and Sabin poliovirus vaccines. Jonas Salk developed a killed viral vaccine in the mid-1950s that is given by injection. A few years later, Albert Sabin devised an oral vaccine consisting of live but weakened polioviruses. OPV is administered orally, mimicking natural poliovirus infection.

Typhoid is another example where attenuated and inactivated vaccines are available. Live, oral cholera vaccines will most likely be available within a few years. Among veterinary vaccines, killed and live, attenuated rabies vaccines are available. According to conventional wisdom, live vaccines induce more persistent immunity, although there are exceptions to this rule.[7]

Toxoids vs Vaccines

A vaccine is a formulation of whole or fractional microorganisms (eg, bacteria, viruses) or portions of them. Toxoids are a subset of vaccines. Toxoids are formed by inactivating a biological toxin, usually by mixing it with formaldehyde. Toxoids retain the ability to stimulate antitoxin formation (eg, specific antibodies against the natural toxin).

DTP provides examples of both because it is a combination of diphtheria and tetanus toxoids plus pertussis vaccine. The toxoids cause recipients to manufacture their own antidiphtheria and antitetanus antitoxin antibodies. Antitoxins have no direct effect on the *Corynebacterium diphtheriae* and *Clostridium tetani* bacteria themselves. Antibiotics are needed to eradicate them. Pertussis vaccine induces antibodies directed against pertussis bacteria. Because toxoids are a special kind of vaccine, it is proper simply to refer to DTP as a vaccine.

Several other vaccine formulations are available in the tetanus-diphtheria family that deserve discussion. Diphtheria and tetanus toxoids are available in two different combinations: The full-strength product (DT) is used for children $<$ 7 years old; a vaccine with a lower concentration of diphtheria toxoid (Td) protects people ≥ 7 years old with fewer side effects. When recommending vaccines, these rules can be helpful:

1.) DTP is preferred over DT for children < 7 years old except for rare contraindications to pertussis vaccine;
2.) Td is preferred over tetanus toxoid (TT) alone, so people do not become susceptible to diphtheria;
3.) the adsorbed form of TT is preferred over the fluid form because it yields higher antibody concentrations.[7]

Polysaccharide vs Proteinaceous Vaccines

Polysaccharide vaccines contain sugar fragments purified from the capsules of certain bacteria. Protein vaccines consist of proteins found inside or on the surface of bacteria or viruses. For example, influenza vaccines rely on protein constituents while pneumococcal vaccines consist of capsular polysaccharides. Protein vaccines generally induce immunity of longer duration than polysaccharide vaccines. Compared with protein antigens, T-cell memory response to booster doses of polysaccharide vaccines is reduced in young children or in immunodeficient hosts.

In contrast with protein vaccines, polysaccharide vaccines (eg, Hib, meningococcal, pneumococcal) are T-cell independent immunogens, which induce a T-cell effect. T-helper lymphocytes regulate maturation, differentiation and proliferation of antibody-producing B-cell subpopulations. Children < 2 years of age do not respond as well to polysaccharide vaccines as they do to proteinaceous ones. Protein-based vaccines work in very young infants.

This situation is well illustrated in the history of *Haemophilus influenzae* type b vaccines. The initial Hib vaccines, licensed in the US beginning in April 1985, contained polysaccharides only. This limited them to use in children ≥ 24 months of age. Later, when scientists developed methods of linking or conjugating these polysaccharides to protein carriers, immunization of children ≥ 2 months of age became possible. These second-generation Hib vaccines, first licensed in December 1987, contain the same polysaccharides as the original Hib vaccines. The combination of polysaccharide and protein increases antibody responses in infants by inducing a T-cell response.[7]

Human vs Animal Antibodies

Rabies immune globulin (RIG) harvested from human serum and equine antirabies serum (ARS) harvested from horses are effective in the prevention of rabies. RIG has entirely replaced ARS in the US and Canada because giving human immune globulins to human patients causes far fewer side effects (eg, hypersensitivity, serum sickness) than giving antibodies harvested from animals.[7]

Another consideration is that animal, or heterologous, IgG has a shorter biological half-life in humans. Its half-life ranges from 8 to 15 days, compared with 23 days for human IgG. Thus, passive immunization with animal antibodies protects for a shorter interval than human antibodies. For these reasons, equine tetanus antitoxin has been replaced by human tetanus immune globulin (TIG).

Drug Interactions

Vaccines and antibodies are drugs, therefore, it is reasonable to expect that drug interactions might affect clinical performance. This section relates several general principles about immunologic drug interactions. More information about immunologic drug interactions, including comprehensive tables, is provided in *ImmunoFacts: Vaccines & Immunologic Drugs.*[7]

Antibody Interference: Inactivated vaccines can be given at any time before or after administration of antibody products. Live vaccines, especially measles or varicella vaccines, should be given 2 weeks before or 2 to 11 months after antibody products, depending on the antibody dose administered. If a shorter interval is used, revaccinate after the proper interval or check the antibody concentration and revaccinate if needed.[9-10]

Simultaneity: There is one general contraindication to the simultaneous administration of vaccines. Giving cholera and yellow-fever vaccines simultaneously will reduce the antibody response to both vaccines. Separate immunization with these vaccines by 3 or more weeks if possible. Observe the following intervals for other vaccines if they are not given simultaneously:[9,11]

• Two inactivated vaccines:	no minimum, any interval acceptable
• An inactivated and alive vaccine:	no minimum, any interval acceptable
• Two live vaccines:	4-week minimum between immunizations. This restriction does not apply to intervals for MMR – OPV or OPV – oral typhoid. Any interval is acceptable for those combinations.

Immunosuppression: Administration of inactivated or live bacterial or viral vaccines to immunosuppressed people may not result in an adequate response to immunization. Inactivated vaccines are not a hazard to immunosuppressed people, but vaccine efficacy may be substantially reduced. Immunization with live bacterial or viral vaccines in immunosuppressed people is generally contraindicated because of the risk of vaccine-induced infection. In either case, these individuals may remain susceptible to infection despite having received an appropriate vaccination. If feasible, measure specific serum antibody concentrations or other immunologic response at an appropriate interval after immunization to assess immunity.[7,9]

Subunit vs Whole Vaccines

Next, we will consider immunopharmaceutics, the study of the characteristics of immunologic dosage forms and immunologic drug delivery.[12]

Microbial vaccines can be produced either from whole microorganisms or subunits of those organisms. A well-known example is the dichotomy between split-virion and whole-virion influenza vaccines. The split vaccine consists of chemically disrupted viruses. The smaller viral particle size of split vaccines reduces the incidence of adverse reactions (eg, fever) in children. Whole-virus vaccine is composed of intact, albeit inactivated, viruses. Modern split- and whole-virus influenza vaccines are immunogenic to an equal extent.[7]

Tradition has a great deal to do with why a whole-virus vaccine is produced. Until the early 1970s, influenza vaccines were calibrated in chick-cell agglutinating (CCA) units. At that time, whole vaccines were thought to be more immunogenic in children although more reactogenic than their split-virion counterparts. The effect was most notable in unprimed people. Current influenza vaccines are standardized by the more reliable immunodiffusion method, which measures the actual mass of antigen. This change is thought to remove any significant difference in efficacy between the two formulations.

The pertussis component of DTP offers another well-known example where two different forms of vaccine are available. The traditional DTP vaccine (now called DTwP) contains whole-cell pertussis vaccine: whole pertussis bacteria killed with formaldehyde. Beginning in December 1991, the FDA licensed DTP vaccines containing acellular pertussis components (called DTaP). Acellular pertussis vaccines contain only certain fragments of pertussis bacteria. The presence of fewer pertussis proteins is believed to give DTaP vaccines their advantage of causing fewer bothersome side effects.

Other vaccines are now, or have previously been, available in subunit form. Hepatitis B vaccine is a purified preparation of the hepatitis B surface antigen to where protective antibodies develop. Rabies vaccines are whole-virion products although split-virion vaccines have been available at other times. Polysaccharides obviously constitute only a part of the bacteria.

Solutions vs Suspension

Two forms of tetanus toxoid are available in the US: Fluid and adsorbed dosage forms. Adsorption is giving tetanus toxoid complexed with aluminum phosphate or aluminum hydroxide; this induces a stronger response than a true solution of tetanus toxoid. The antigen-alum complexes more readily mobilize macrophages.[7,13]

The only product for which a choice is currently available between fluid (eg, solution) and adsorbed (eg, suspension) forms is tetanus toxoid. Both products induce adequate immunity response, but a dose of alum-adsorbed suspension elicits higher antitoxin concentrations. Higher concentrations lead to more persistent antitoxin levels than the fluid form.

CDC guidelines do not mention single-antigen tetanus toxoid. Combined tetanus and diphtheria toxoids are adsorbed formulations in either pediatric or adult concentrations and are the proper agents for standard wound prophylaxis. The only rational remaining use of fluid tetanus toxoid is when diluted as a delayed-hypersensitivity reagent.

Standard vs Hyperimmune Antibodies

Immune globulins are concentrated solutions of antibodies. They are frequently used for passive immunization or to treat certain immunodeficiencies. They attack infections in a specific (eg, neutralization) and nonspecific (eg, induction of complement) manner. Efficacy for many indications depends on the specificity of the antibody in the product.

Consider the dichotomy between broad-spectrum IGIM and hepatitis B immune globulin (HBIG). Immune globulin intramuscular (IGIM) is useful against measles and hepatitis A because the pool of volunteer blood donors from which it is harvested has high concentrations of antibodies against these and other microbes. Most lots of IGIM have little activity against hepatitis B virus because the pool has little of this specific antibody. Conversely, HBIG is a hyperimmune product with a known level of biological activity against the hepatitis B virus. HBIG is harvested from people with high HBIG concentrations.

To help assure broad-spectrum efficacy, each lot of IGIM requires a serum pool of at least 1000 donors. IGIM harvested in the US has little demonstrable activity against yellow-fever virus because few in the volunteer pool have been exposed to this microbe or its vaccine. Batches of immune globulins available in the US vary in their activity against unevenly distributed infectious agents (eg, cytomegalovirus, Epstein-Barr virus). Some manufacturers have responded to clinicians' requests for product labeling with specific activity against a litany of microorganisms to guide anti-infective therapy. These manufacturers are willing to provide lot-specific information about specific antibody concentrations of a given production batch.

Hyperimmune globulins can either be produced by assembling volunteer donors who have large quantities of the desired antibody, by screening units of blood about to expire (eg, CMV-IG) or by intentionally hyperimmunizing volunteers to a specific antigen.

Equine antitoxins and antivenins are hyperimmune immune globulins in the sense that they are high-titer antibody products that neutralize certain toxins or venoms. The horses are intentionally exposed to the toxins or venoms so that the equine antibodies could later be harvested and processed into drugs for human use.

Production Methods

Source materials and production methods can have real and imagined effects on the immunologic drugs produced. Consider the dichotomy between the original hepatitis B vaccine (*Heptavax-B,* Merck) and the two current vaccines (Merck's *Recombivax-HB* and SmithKline Beecham's *Engerix-B*). *Heptavax-B* was produced using the purified plasma donated by human volunteers who were infected with hepatitis B virus. Despite scientific evidence to the contrary, many people feared disease transmission from the source plasma used for *Heptavax-B.* The other two vaccines are manufactured by collecting hepatitis B surface antigen (HBsAg) produced by yeast cells modified by recombinant-DNA biotechnology. Clinical data show the two source types (plasma and yeast) to be comparably effective in immunoprophylaxis.[7]

Other source differences exist or existed for rubella and rabies vaccines. The HPV-77 and Cendehill strains of attenuated rubella virus were originally produced in dog-kidney, duck-embryo or rabbit-kidney media. The current RA 27/3 strain is grown in human diploid cell culture. Early rabies vaccines were variously produced in mouse brain or duck-embryo media.

Nerve-tissue rabies vaccines (NTVs) had a high adverse-reaction rate and provided incomplete protection. The current rabies vaccines are grown either in human diploid cell or diploid fetal-rhesus lung culture media. NTVs required 23 doses compared with 14 doses for duck-embryo vaccines and five doses for modern vaccines.[7]

Production processes vary among the drugs produced from elements of human blood. For example, IGIV is prepared by the Cohn-Oncley cold-ethanol fractionation process. This process inactivates most viruses, including the HIV and HBV. Recently, solvent-detergent treatment or other virucidal steps have been required for manufacturing any immune globulin product. Virucidal treatment is important to inactivate lipid-enveloped viruses (eg, hepatitis C). Heat treatment of alpha1-proteinase inhibitor (*Prolastin,* Bayer) used in the management of congenital panacinar emphysema does not completely eliminate hepatitis B virus transmission. Hepatitis B immunization is recommended for people expected to receive *Prolastin.*[7]

The differences in clinical significance of these and other production processes has not been completely defined. It is differences like those discussed above that make regulation and standardization of biological drugs more intricate than chemical drugs.

Preferred vs Inadequate Diluents

Diluents are important for reconstituting powdered drugs and for compounding dilutions for hypersensitivity testing and immunotherapy. Sterile diluents are available variously in 1.8, 4, 4.5, 9, 30 ml and 100 ml vials. Manufacturers and resellers include the manufacturers of allergen extracts.[7,16]

Diluents are not equally effective at preserving the potency of their active ingredients. Aqueous allergen extracts, such as *Hymenoptera* venoms, are commonly diluted with a solution containing 0.03% human serum albumin (HSA) as a protein preservative, 0.9% sodium chloride for isotonicity and 0.4% phenol as an antimicrobial agent.

Dilution with 50% glycerin in sterile water provides a higher degree of protein preservation than HSA, but glycerin injections may cause local irritation or sterile abscesses. Glycerin is often used as the diluent for prick skin-test dilutions because the viscosity of the glycerin retards the flow of one prick-test reagent into neighboring reagents. Glycerin may increase the incidence of false-positive skin-test reactions especially in the higher dose associated with ID injection. Injections > 0.2 ml of a 50% glycerin product may be painful. Concentrations of sterile parenteral glycerin, ranging from 10% to 95%, are commercially available.

Isotonic 0.9% sodium chloride can serve as an effective diluent, although dilutions are not stable for more than several hours or days. The presence of preservatives (eg, thimerosal, phenol) in sodium chloride diluents generally poses no problems except in the exceptional patient who may be hypersensitive to the preservative. "Phenol-saline" (0.9% sodium chloride with 0.4% phenol) (eg, *Allpyral, Center-Al)* is the preferred diluent for alum-precipitated allergen extracts.

Differential Utilization

Clinical Goal: Clinicians employ immunologic drugs to serve a wide range of purposes including the spectrum of prevention, diagnosis and treatment. Immunologic drugs variously include vaccines, immune globulins, toxoids, antitoxins, venoms, antivenoms, allergens, antigens, interferons, interleukins, colony-stimulating factors, stimulants, suppressants and modifiers.[7,12]

- Prevention: Vaccines, *Hymenoptera* venoms, antibodies, immunoantidotes and similar agents are administered to prevent infection, disease or illness, but the types of prevention vary considerably. Vaccines are used to prevent disease months, years or decades in the future while antibodies are generally used more acutely. Hepatitis B immune globulin (HBIG) is used for prophylaxis in cases of needlestick injury. Rh_o(D) immune globulin prevents disease in subsequent offspring of the recipient.
- Diagnosis: Immunologic drugs are used in the detection of infections (eg, tuberculin), the diagnosis of allergy (eg, allergen extracts, benzylpenicilloyl polylysine) or other diseases (eg, a radiolabeled antibody), the staging of a disease (eg, anergy tests for HIV) or the assessment of general immune function (eg, anergy tests).[7]
- Treatment: Immunotherapy may include IGIV, an antitoxin, an antivenin, an allergen extract, digoxin Fab, an interferon, or a colony-stimulating factor.[7]
- Multiple Uses: Some immunologic drugs are used in several modes either alternatively or simultaneously. Post-exposure rabies vaccination can be construed as prevention of rabies disease or as presumptive treatment of rabies infection. Several products can be used for distinctly different purposes depending on the case. The various anti-lymphocyte immune globulins can be used either for prevention or treatment of acute organ-rejection episodes. BCG vaccine can be used for prevention of tuberculosis or for treatment of certain bladder cancers. Tetanus toxoid is useful either in inducing antitoxin antibodies or diluted as an intradermal test to assess anergy. Pre-exposure hepatitis B vaccine is an example of primary prevention, while post-exposure vaccination is a form of secondary prevention.

Vaccination Policy-Making

National vaccine schedules and policies for the US are developed by a variety of experts. The Advisory Committee on Immunization Practices (ACIP) and the Centers for Disease Control & Prevention (CDC) are the nation's preeminent authorities. The next major source is the Committee on Infectious Diseases of the American Academy of Pediatrics (AAP), whose published report is known as the "Red Book." Other expert groups include the Adult Immunization Task Force of the American College of Physicians (ACP) and a similar group at the American Academy of Family Physicians (AAFP).[17-20]

The FDA determines which new vaccines and antibodies have sufficient evidence of safety and efficacy to warrant a license. The FDA is aided in these evaluations by its Vaccines & Related Biological Products Advisory Committee (VRBAC) and other advisory committees.

Changes in immunization policy are being published with increasing frequency. In the decade before 1985, the nation's childhood immunization schedule remained virtually unchanged. Since 1985, major changes have been adopted at least annually. The future is likely to be similarly full of changes. It is important for all professionals to stay up-to-date, using frequently updated references, such as *ImmunoFacts: Vaccines & Immunologic Drugs.*[7]

All vs Some People

A nation's immunization policies for available vaccines vary according to many factors including the epidemiology of the diseases involved, the immunologic characteristics of the vaccines, the sociologic characteristics of clients and clinicians, the structure of the healthcare infrastructure, the likelihood and consequences of adverse effects and the costs associated with each factor. Public health officials may recommend one of several delivery strategies to combat vaccine-preventable infections. The two main approaches are universal coverage or targeting of high-risk groups.[12,17]

For some vaccines, universal vaccination of a whole population is recommended (eg, Hib). In some cases, immunization is so important to society that it is mandated before employment or admission into schools or nursing homes. All infants or children, with exceedingly few exceptions, should be immunized against diphtheria; tetanus; pertussis (DTP); poliovirus; Hib; hepatitis B; measles, mumps, rubella (MMR) and varicella. This is a strategy of universal immunization of the population.

Certain subgroups may be identified whose risk of infection, disease or death is higher than the norm. For example, we do not recommend rabies immunization for the entire US population, but we do recommend it for veterinarians and veterinary students. Similarly, hepatitis B vaccine is recommended for healthcare workers with potential contact with blood or body fluids. Influenza and pneumococcal vaccines are especially encouraged for people with heart disease, lung disease or diabetes and those ≥ 65 years of age even if otherwise healthy. Immunizations for international travel are another example of targeting those likely to be exposed to unusual microbes (eg, yellow fever, Japanese encephalitis, typhoid).

Recommendations for hepatitis B vaccine changed in 1992 from select use in people potentially exposed to body fluids to a dual strategy of targeted immunization for high-risk groups and universal vaccination of all American children and adolescents. Among adults, special efforts are made to assess pregnant and postpartum women for immunity to rubella.

Experts at the Centers for Disease Control & Prevention list several groups who most need influenza vaccine and then add the following subset: "Any person who wishes to reduce the likelihood of becoming ill with influenza."

Before, During or After?

Rabies vaccine may be used for pre-exposure protection of veterinarians and others with predictable risk. Post-exposure rabies prophylaxis is given to people only after they have been bitten or otherwise exposed. Among healthcare workers, it is common practice to emphasize pre-exposure vaccination with hepatitis B vaccine rather than post-exposure "needle-stick" protection with HBIG.

Pre-exposure protection is adopted when exposure can reasonably be predicted. Rabies is a good example where vaccination is an emergency measure to prevent disease, qualifying as an antidote. Vaccination may be recommended after disease to prevent disease recurrence. Children < 24 months old who develop invasive Hib disease do not develop immunity and should still be immunized. Vaccinate anyone with a chronic disease or advancing age who develops pneumonia against influenza and pneumococcal disease.

Process vs Outcome

Sticking a needle into someone's arm and marking an immunization record does not guarantee that the recipient is immune from disease. Even if we go to the trouble to measure an antibody concentration and find it adequate, we cannot be assured of protection.

No prophylactic immunologic drug will protect 100% of recipients against corresponding infections. In addition, several factors beyond the manufacturer's control can reduce the efficacy of an immunologic product or result in an adverse effect from its use. Such factors include improper storage and handling of the product, dosage, method of administration, patient diagnosis and biological and other differences in individuals.

It is proper for clinicians to focus on a patient's health outcome (eg, death, disability, disease) rather than merely working to improve process indicators (eg, laboratory values, culture results) for their own sake. In a strict sense, immunizations are process indicators of the delivery of preventive healthcare. Our current focus on outcomes does not adequately consider how to measure disease avoidance for the individual.

It is appropriate for clinicians to consider vaccinations as surrogate outcomes. If you have received the proper number of doses of measles vaccine, you have taken prudent steps to avoid measles. It has some similarities to taking the prudent steps of buying insurance, brushing your teeth or rust-proofing a car. You have assembled the appropriate defenses.

Of course, it remains for our society's public-health scientists to continually measure the effect of immunization delivery to constantly improve it. To these professionals, the act of vaccination will always remain a process that contributes to the health outcome of a community.

The bottom line in comparing and contrasting the various immunological drugs is equivalence of clinical effect. Any consideration of the differential pharmacology or pharmaceutics of an immunologic drug must address the health outcome of the drug's recipient. Did the vaccine prevent the disease? Did the antibody treat the disease? Did the test detect the disease? Was the patient's care affected by changing brands or sources or types of an immunological drug during prophylaxis, diagnosis or therapy?

The term "therapeutic equivalence" is commonly used to imply comparable clinical effect among chemical drugs. Assessment of some immunologic drugs may require the corollary concepts of prophylactic equivalence or diagnostic equivalence.

For hepatitis B vaccines, the products are prophylactically equivalent (adjusting for the proper dose). For BCG, the two products are not equivalent for prevention of tuberculosis.

Immunologic drugs have many similarities but also many idiosyncrasies. It is every health professional's responsibility to assure that these drugs are used optimally with full understanding of the properties, actions and effects of each agent, to best prevent, diagnose or treat disease.

References

[1] Grabenstein JD. Don't say biologics if you mean *immunologics. Am J Hosp Pharm* 1988;45:1941-2.
[2] Roitt IM, Brostoff J, Male DK. *Immunology,* 4th ed. Baltimore: Mosby, 1996.
[3] Bellanti JA. Basic immunologic principles underlying vaccination procedures. *Pediatr Clin N Amer* 1990;37:513-30.
[4] Stites DP, Terr AI. *Basic & Clinical Immunology,* 7th ed. Norwalk, CT: Appleton & Lange, 1991.
[5] Grabenstein JD. Pharmacoimmunology 102: Comparisons & contrasts. *Hosp Pharm* 1993;28:544-6,548,560.
[6] Koeller J, Tami J, ed. *Concepts in Immunology and Immunotherapeutics,* 2nd ed. Bethesda, MD: American Society of Hospital Pharmacists, 1992.
[7] Grabenstein JD. *ImmunoFacts: Vaccines & Immunologic Drugs.* St. Louis: Facts and Comparisons, May 1997.
[8] McGhee JR, Mestecky J. In defense of mucosal surfaces: Development of novel vaccines for IgA responses protective at the portals of entry of microbial pathogens. *Infect Dis Clin N Amer* 1990;4:315-41.
[9] Advisory Committee on Immunization Practices. General recommendations on immunization. *MMWR* 1994;43(RR-1):1-38.
[10] Grabenstein JD. American immunization policies: Actions speak louder than words. *Hosp Pharm* 1993;28:1233-4,1237-40.
[11] Gizurarson S. Optimal delivery of vaccines: Clinical pharmacokinetic considerations. *Clin Pharmacokinet* 1996;30:1-15.
[12] Grabenstein JD. Pharmacoimmunology 103: Differential pharmaceutics & utilization. *Hosp Pharm* 1993;28:688-91,694,697.
[13] Grabenstein JD. Stop buying tetanus toxoid (with one exception). *Hosp Pharm* 1990;25:361-2.
[14] Stiehm ER. Standard and special human immune serum globulins as therapeutic agents. *Pediatrics* 1979;63:301-19.
[15] Dwyer JM. Thirty years of supplying the missing link: History of gamma globulin therapy for immunodeficient states. *Am J Med* 1984;76:46-52.
[16] Grabenstein JD. Immunologic necessities: Diluents, adjuvants, & excipients. *Hosp Pharm* 1996;31:1387-8,1390,1392,1397-8,1401.
[17] American Academy of Pediatrics. Recommended timing of routine measles immunization for children who have recently received immune globulin preparations. *Pediatrics* 1994;93:682-5.
[18] Hinman AR, Orenstein WA. Public health considerations. In: Plotkin SA, Mortimer EA Jr., ed. *Vaccines,* 2nd ed. Philadelphia: WB Saunders, 1994:903-32.
[19] American College of Physicians. *Guide for Adult Immunization,* 3rd ed. Philadelphia: American College of Physicians, 1994.
[20] Peter G, ed. *1994 Red Book: Report of the Committee on Infectious Diseases,* 23rd ed. Elk Grove Village, IL: American Academy of Pediatrics, 1994.

CHAPTER 4

Making Vaccine Decisions

Sociologists recognize five key factors in a person's decision whether or not to be vaccinated:[1-3]

- Perceived susceptibility to a disease
- Perceived seriousness of a disease
- Perceived vaccine barriers (eg, side effects, access)
- Perceived vaccine benefits
- Social influence from a pharmacist, nurse or physician.

This chapter will review the appropriate techniques to identify people who need to be vaccinated and discuss how to motivate them to receive vaccination.

Nearly everyone believes that they are susceptible to rabies (if bitten) and that rabies is a serious disease. This begins to explain why rabies is the only overused immunization in America. Fewer people believe that influenza is serious, but reminding them that influenza and pneumonia are the sixth leading cause of death in the US can help put things in perspective.

The death toll and disease from vaccine-preventable diseases was presented in an earlier chapter. Remember that the following groups of people most need vaccines. This list starts with the greatest causes of death and disease and follows a descending sequence:

- Adults and people with chronic diseases at risk for influenza and pneumococcal pneumonia, especially those ≥ 65 years of age.
- Adults, adolescents and children at risk for hepatitis B.
- Children delayed in receiving sufficient doses of diphtheria-tetanus-pertussis (DTP), measles-mumps-rubella (MMR), *Haemophilus influenzae* type b (Hib), poliovirus and varicella vaccines.
- Adults and adolescents needing immunization against diphtheria, tetanus, measles, mumps, rubella, Hib, poliovirus or varicella.

Finding Those Who Need Vaccines

Methods of identifying a person's immunization needs can be organized in several ways. A model screening form has been included in chapter seven on "Immunization Documentation." Clinicians can be involved in some or all of the following forms of immunization surveillance:[4]

- *Occurrence screening* identifies vaccine needs at the time of particular events. These include hospital or nursing home admissions, discharges, ambulatory or emergency room visits, mid-decade birthdays (years 25, 35, 45, etc.) and any time anyone contacts the health-care delivery system.
- *Diagnosis screening* reviews vaccine needs among patients with conditions that place them at increased risk of preventable infections. Diagnoses such as hemophilia, thalassemia, most cancers, sickle-cell

anemia, chronic alcoholism, cirrhosis, cerebrospinal fluid leaks, HIV infection, multiple antibiotic allergies and other disorders should prompt attention to a patient's vaccine needs.

- *Procedure screening* identifies vaccine needs based on medical or surgical procedures. These include splenectomy, heart or lung surgery, organ transplant, chemotherapy, radiation therapy, immunosuppression of other types, dialysis and prescription of certain medications.[5]
- *Periodic mass screening* can be conducted during autumn influenza programs and during programs to control outbreaks (eg, local measles or pertussis epidemics). Schools, nursing homes and other institutions can perform such screening when registering new cohorts of students, residents or other groups. Mass screening also may be appropriate where no comprehensive immunization program has been conducted in the past few years. Mass screenings help improve vaccine-coverage rates quickly, but long-term benefits are much greater when such intermittent programs are combined with ongoing, comprehensive screening efforts.

Once you identify people needing immunization, advise them of their infection risk and encourage them to receive the immunizations they need. If appropriate, remind the corresponding physicians of their patients' need for vaccination. Do not reschedule people needing immunizations to a future appointment that may be missed. Rather, vaccinate them during the current healthcare contact unless valid contraindications exist. In general, mild fevers or mild diarrheal illness do not contraindicate immunization nor do current antimicrobial therapy, convalescence, prematurity, pregnancy, recent exposure to an infectious disease, breast-feeding, history of nonspecific allergies or family histories of allergies, convulsions, sudden infant death syndrome or adverse events following vaccination.

Advising people of their need for immunization can take several forms. In ambulatory settings, individualized or form letters or postcards can be mailed, people can be telephoned or an insert can be included with bills, reminders or prescriptions informing people of their infection risk and the availability and efficacy of vaccines. For nursing home clients, communication with the clients' family members is important.

Adhesive warning labels can be affixed to prescription containers for drugs that indicate need for vaccination against influenza and pneumonia (eg, digoxin, warfarin, theophylline, insulin). These labels would be analogous to labels currently in widespread use (eg, "shake well," "take with food or milk"). Such labels might read "You May Need Flu or Pneumonia Vaccine: Ask Your Doctor or Pharmacist." For inpatients and institutional residents, chart notes, consultations, messages to patients or family and similar means can be used.

While many of the screening criteria described above will focus on candidates for influenza or pneumococcal vaccines, conduct comprehensive screening on the individuals identified this way. While assessing these patients, take the opportunity to check for vaccine needs: Influenza, pneumococcal, or hepatitis B vaccine, tetanus-diphtheria boosters, etc.

How To Motivate Vaccine Candidates

More than 50,000 deaths from vaccine-preventable infections occur in the US per year. Although immunization programs for school-aged children have helped substantially reduce vaccine-preventable diseases, significant morbidity and mortality from these infections continue to occur. These avoidable diseases strike infants, children, adolescents, adults and the elderly. Pharmacists, nurses and physicians are in excellent positions to counsel individuals about this type of disease prevention, given their knowledge of immunizations and access to people at risk.

Through effective interviewing and counseling, pharmacists, nurses and physicians can increase vaccine acceptance. The only way to determine a person's vaccine needs is to question and evaluate that person's health risks. An effective interview can be conducted in 1 to 5 minutes. Solicit pertinent information regarding medical and immunization history, then use this information in deciding which vaccines the person needs.[6]

Motivation is the second step: Educating people to change their immunization behavior. Effective motivation of any type requires that you provide information customized to that person's individual needs. Conduct the education in an understandable manner, appropriate for the person's level of understanding. This will enable the person to accept and carry out the vaccine recommendations. In this regard, counseling about vaccines is not much different from counseling people about other medications.

This section will review a model of health behavior and discuss three phases used in teaching and counseling people; effective questioning techniques will be reviewed. These concepts will be cited in specific interchanges between professional and patient for disease prevention and appropriate vaccination.

Model of Health Behavior

The reasons people act to prevent disease can be explained via a respected paradigm called the Health Belief Model. Not surprisingly, a person's perceptions of susceptibility to and severity of a given disease, perceived benefits of acting and perceived barriers to taking action are the most frequently cited explanations of someone's health behavior.[8-10]

In general, people who are unconcerned with an aspect of their health are unlikely to perceive problems or act to improve their health. If the person sees no value in following a treatment or prevention plan, then recommendations will probably not be adopted. Showing friendliness and receptivity, providing justification of the prevention strategy and exerting medical authority concerning possible long-term benefits gained through intervention have all been shown to increase motivation. Motivation may vary over time and should be reevaluated occasionally.

Other variables that contribute to health behavior include the person's readiness to act and the extent to which a person believes an action will reduce a threat. The person's perceptions of disease susceptibility and vaccine efficacy may not correspond with scientifically accepted fact. Education provided by health experts is very important.

Barriers to vaccination include factors such as fear, anxiety, inconvenience, pain and expense. If the person considers barriers to be relatively weak and his or her readiness to be vaccinated is great, then he or she is likely to accept immunization. Conversely, if the person's readiness is low and the barriers are strong, then the desired behavior is less likely to occur.[8,10]

Often, you will be talking with the person's agent. For example, parents make immunization decisions for their children and many adult children assist with immunization decisions for their aging parents. Viewing the immunization decision through the eyes of the decision maker is important. The key elements in a person's immunization decision are perceptions of disease susceptibility and severity, barriers and vaccine efficacy. Knowing this, you are well on your way to influencing decision-making processes regarding immunizations.

Immunization costs are only a minor barrier to most people. More serious obstacles are limited places and times of vaccine availability. Consider a set of parents with all good intentions to immunize their children. They may have to take time off from a minimum-wage job, ride a bus or two across town to the public clinic, wait an hour or more to be seen and repeat this procedure at least four times between birth and 6 years of age for each child. Under these conditions, it is easy to see how immunization delivery rates may lag behind recommendations.

Most people believe that vaccines work or else they are easily persuaded when offered the facts. Nonetheless, some myths persist, such as "Oh, I always get the flu from a flu shot." Explaining the manufacturing method of mixing influenza viruses with formaldehyde can help dispel this myth.

Perhaps the most important contribution someone can make is simply informing the person or parent of disease risk, then encourage immunization at any of several locations as soon as possible. Experience from a variety of settings show that 50% to 75% or more will act based on a professional's vaccine recommendation.

INTERVIEWING PEOPLE ABOUT IMMUNIZATIONS

Phase I: Assessment

During the initial phase of the immunization interview, determine whether the person has risk factors that warrant vaccination. Find out how fully the person understands his or her risk of infection and the benefits and risks of vaccines. Ask about infection risk factors based on age, occupation, lifestyle, underlying disease states and other factors.[6,11] A summary of vaccine indications organized by age, risk factors and other important variables is printed in chapter two on "Too Much Disease, Too Many Deaths." An immunization screening form that allows individual assessment of indications and contraindications for vaccination appears in chapter seven on "Immunization Documentation."

By using several different types of questions, you can prompt people to share their understanding of disease risk and vaccine efficacy. The vaccine candidate is the best single source of information. The assessment phase also gives the vaccine candidate an opportunity to form an opinion of the sincerity and credibility of the person doing the motivating.

Questioning techniques used in the assessment phase gathers information about the person's medication history, allergies, immunization status, underlying disease states, fears and perception of susceptibility. General questions regarding person immunization history are suggested on the next page. Identifying which vaccines this individual needs permits you to start developing a plan for the person to implement.

Several references provide detailed information about vaccines used or available in other countries. *ImmunoFacts: Vaccines & Immunologic Drugs* lists vaccines available abroad by generic and proprietary names and immunologic terms in several languages.[4]

Types of Questions to Ask

Using open-ended questions allows you to assess a person's understanding of his or her risk of infection and the value of immunizations. Open-ended questions are helpful if you want more information from the person's point of view. This type of query allows the interviewee maximum freedom to describe things. Examples include inquiries such as "Describe your family records for immunizations," or "Tell me about any serious vaccine reactions you had in the past." Open-ended questions avoid potential bias on the interviewer's part and allow responses without restriction.[6-7,12]

Another approach helpful in interviewing and motivation is the use of reflective questions. This type encourages broader communication and helps the person explain earlier statements. You can gain a better understanding of the person's concerns and perspectives. Examples include "If you had a choice, would you rather prevent an infection or treat it?" or "Do you worry about the flu?"

Specifier questions can be used to ask for detailed information. This type addresses implications in generalizations or unclear statements. Examples include "Do you have records of your entire family's immunizations or just the children?" and "Are you allergic to tetanus toxoid or tetanus antitoxin? These questions allow the person to respond with full detail and description.

Use justifying questions sparingly. This question type encourages the person to explain reasons, attitudes or feelings. "What makes you think that flu shots cause the flu?" is an example of a justifying inquiry. These questions can provide the person an opportunity to think and reason through a situation.

Directive questions are useful if you want to limit possible answers and guide the conversation in a particular direction. An example is "Have you ever been exposed to blood or blood products?"

The last category that can be used in interviews is the hypothetical question. This query presents a possibility or suggestion to open a discussion, or it can lead the person toward a conclusion, such as "What would happen to your family if you were hospitalized because of influenza or pneumonia?"

Here are some ways to ask about immunization status:

1.) Are you aware that you may be susceptible to ______________?
2.) Have you ever been vaccinated against ______________ before?
3.) When did you receive your last dose of ______________ vaccine?
4.) What makes you reluctant to get ______________ vaccine?
5.) Are there barriers that prevent or discourage you from becoming vaccinated (for example: cost, travel, fear)?
6.) Are you aware of any allergies or previous adverse reactions you have had to vaccines?
7.) When were you (your children) last vaccinated?
8.) When are you (your family) scheduled for your next vaccines?

Additional questions may be appropriate in certain settings.

Types of Questions to Avoid

There are several types of questions to avoid in interviewing a person. One example is the closed-ended question because it does not allow for active information exchange. Closed-ended questions allow only a yes or no response from the person, such as "Are all of your immunizations up to date?" A more effective way to address this topic might be to ask "When did you receive a vaccine most recently? What was it for?" or "When are your next immunizations due?"[6]

Minimize suggestive or leading inquiries; this type tends to propose the desired response within the question itself. It often reflects the opinions of the person asking the questions. A question such as "Did the vaccine make you feel sick?" can lead the person to respond with an affirmative answer. It may represent more of your thinking than the true feelings of the person in front of you. One exception might be in taking a person's history of prior tetanus immunization. "Have you been treated in an emergency room in the last few years where you may have received a tetanus booster?" can be helpful in interviewing. Leading questions can be useful to test how closely you both agree. Overall, this type of question tends to bias answers.

Active Listening

Because most people are better senders of information than receivers, be sure to concentrate on the listening component of communication. Good listeners pay close attention and keep open views about what the other person is saying. Patience contributes to good listening. Let the interviewee know there is ample time to discuss any issue. To enhance active listening, use paraphrasing and summation to highlight key points. Health professionals who are effective listeners are more likely to interpret the person's message accurately.[13-15]

An important role for the immunization counselor is to dispel misconceptions and misinformation about vaccines. For example, be prepared to counter common misconceptions about influenza vaccine with facts about its safety and low incidence of side effects. Comparably, the risks of encephalopathy following pertussis vaccine are recognized to be much lower than earlier thought if there is any causal link at all. Whenever you find yourself confronted with side-effect disputes, ask if the risk of side effects does or does not outweigh the risk of the disease to be prevented.

Screening for Vaccine Needs

Included in this book are two helpful tools. Nearby is a list of key questions to ask before immunizing. Include these seven questions in any immunization program you conduct. The second tool provided is the basis for a screening form you can develop for your practice site. It appears in chapter seven on "Immunization Documentation." The form is annotated with comments for responding to the vaccine candidate's answers. An immunization-screening form is appropriate for:

- Assessing the immunization needs of clients of private physicians and public health clinics
- Assessing the immunization needs of people admitted to a hospital or an emergency room or entering nursing homes, schools or other institutions
- Assessing employees' immunization needs, helping immunization programs run by occupational-health personnel
- Screening people for vaccination during influenza seasons or other infectious outbreaks (eg, measles, pertussis).

Although the form is designed to consider pediatric patients as well as adults, it is not specifically designed for well-baby screening. Another more specific form may be appropriate in such cases.

Most significantly, this form allows *individual* assessment of someone's indications and contraindications for vaccination. Using this instrument can turn what would have been a mass vaccination program into many individualized immunization encounters. It serves as a summary of immunization history to date, as well as a record of immunizations ordered and given during that day's immunization assessment.

As automation of patient medical records becomes more prevalent, enter immunization data into automated medical records. For example, "smart cards" that record the patient's diagnoses, current medications, laboratory values and other pertinent information should record the patient's immunization history.

Key Questions to Ask Before Immunizing

1.) Has this person ever had a severe reaction to any vaccine that required medical care? If yes, describe. Immediate, anaphylactic, life-threatening reactions to vaccine components generally bar further vaccinations with a product containing that component. Other reactions are largely irrelevant. See detailed references.

2.) Does this person have a severe fever, diarrhea or vomiting today? If the clinical state is sufficient to refer the person to the next higher level of care (eg, hospitalization, referral to a specialist), defer vaccination until the acute event stabilizes; then vaccinate promptly. Make notes on whose immunizations have been deferred, so you can remind them to resume their immunizations.

3.) a. Is this person or anyone in this home receiving chemotherapy, radiation therapy? Do they have HIV infection, AIDS or any immune disorder?
b. Is there any form of immunosuppression in a potential vaccine recipient or member of the household? If the answer to either 3-a or 3-b is yes, be cautious with use of live vaccines. For example, IPV may be preferred over OPV in these settings.
4.) Has this person received blood or antibodies (immune globulins) in the past 3 to 11 months? If so, be cautious with live vaccines. Timing between antibodies and vaccination depends on the dose of antibody given.
5.) Is this person pregnant or planning pregnancy in the next 3 months? If so, be cautious with live vaccines. Inactivated vaccines are generally safe in pregnancy and may be important to protect the woman's health.

For Childhood Vaccines:

6.) Is this child being evaluated for seizures? If so, withhold pertussis vaccine until the clinical condition stabilizes.
7.) Did this child have any of the following problems within 7 days of earlier vaccines:
   - Fever of 105°F or more
   - Seizures or convulsions
   - Continuous crying for 3 or more hours
   - Unusual sleepiness
   - Unusual, high-pitched scream
   - Collapse or unresponsiveness?

Additional questions may be appropriate in certain settings.

Inappropriate Contraindications: Frequent Misconceptions

People do not like to get injections. This reluctance is perfectly reasonable even if pain is outweighed by the protection conferred by the immunization. Unfortunately, hesitation over injections spurs some people to search for reasons why the injection may be unnecessary.[16-17]

Be wary when evaluating claims of contraindications. Separate true discriminators from spurious ones. If someone erroneously claims an exception, that person will go unvaccinated and remain vulnerable to infection. Not only will that person be personally susceptible, but he or she can aid the spread of an outbreak, putting many at risk.

Explain that exemptions to immunization must be minimized to the fewest possible for personal and societal reasons. A list of inappropriate contraindications appears in the accompanying table. It was derived from a list developed by experts at the CDC. Do NOT routinely withhold immunization in the following instances:

1.) Reaction to a previous dose of diphtheria and tetanus toxoids with pertussis vaccine (DTP) that involved only soreness, redness or swelling in the immediate vicinity of the vaccination site or temperature $< 40.5°C$ ($< 105°F$)

2.) Mild acute illness with low-grade fever or mild diarrheal illness in an otherwise well child
3.) Current antimicrobial therapy or convalescent phase of illness
4.) Prematurity. The appropriate age to initiate immunization of the premature infant is the usual chronologic age from birth. Do not reduce vaccine doses for preterm infants.
5.) Pregnancy in the person or a household contact
6.) Recent exposure to an infectious disease
7.) Breast-feeding. The only vaccine virus that has been isolated from breast milk is rubella vaccine virus. There is no evidence that milk from women immunized against rubella harms infants.
8.) History of nonspecific allergies or allergic relatives
9.) Allergies to penicillin or any other antibiotic, except anaphylactic reactions to neomycin (pertinent for MMR-containing vaccines) or streptomycin (pertinent for oral polio vaccine). No vaccine available in the US or Canada contains penicillin.
10.) Allergies to duck meat or duck feathers. No vaccine available in the US or Canada uses duck products during manufacturing.
11.) A family history of convulsions in people considered for pertussis or measles vaccination
12.) A family history of sudden infant death syndrome (SIDS) in children considered for DTP vaccination
13.) A family history of an adverse event following vaccination unrelated to immunosuppression.

To this list, we add these suggestions. No child should be denied pertussis vaccination without good justification. Do not choose DT over DTP unless CDC criteria are met.

Exercise prudence in assessing claims of allergies that preclude immunization. What reaction did the person have? How long ago? Why does the person believe the reaction and the vaccine are linked? The long-held concerns about egg allergies are being reevaluated as overly restrictive. At any rate, if the person does not develop laryngeal edema or other true allergic symptoms upon eating eggs, give the vaccine. Sensitivity to thimerosal in contact-lens solutions is not sufficient grounds to withhold immunization. Other issues regarding vaccine components are discussed in chapter five on "Special Situations."

With claims of tetanus allergy, differentiate between tetanus antitoxin (where a reaction may have been caused by equine serum) and tetanus toxoid (where a reaction might be caused by too many doses of toxoid). The former is common and the latter is unusual.

If the person is not ill enough to refer to a physician or hospital, the person can be vaccinated. Fever does not adequately reflect severity of illness in children. Minor illnesses (eg, low-grade fever, upper respiratory infection, otitis media, mild diarrhea) are no cause for deferring vaccination.

For hospitalized people, the CDC recommends immunization just before discharge. One exception is that it may be prudent to delay live, attenuated OPV vaccine until after hospital discharge. This helps avoid exposing immunosuppressed people to this virus in an infant's excreta.

No vaccine has ever been shown to be a human teratogen: This includes live rubella virus vaccine for which the wild virus causes horrible birth defects. Inadvertent immunization with a live virus vaccine during pregnancy is not a sufficient cause to terminate pregnancy. Similarly, pregnancy in the household of a potential vaccine recipient is not a reason to delay vaccination with rubella, OPV or varicella vaccines.

People may offer irrational ideas that have no basis in fact. An example might be a claim that a fever or a case of chickenpox is an indication that MMR vaccine failed. It is not possible for someone to develop allergic reactions to products not included in the vaccine (eg, penicillin, bird feathers). A person's history of allergies that are not immediate and life-threatening (eg, anaphylaxis, laryngeal edema) are largely irrelevant.

To close this section, influenza vaccine cannot cause the flu. Influenza viruses are treated with formaldehyde and other chemicals until they are dead, then the remnants are packaged as the vaccine. Some people are incubating an influenza, rhinovirus or adenovirus infection at the time of vaccination that may lead to a coincidental runny nose during the week after vaccination. This coincidence cannot be avoided. Do not blame the vaccine. Other people remember influenza vaccine side effects from the 1960s and 1970s, an era when the vaccines were not as highly purified as they are today. Remind people: Influenza can kill; influenza vaccines save lives.

True and False Contraindications and Precautions[17]

True Contraindications and Precautions	False (Vaccines May Be Administered)
General For All Pediatric Vaccines (DTwP, DTaP, OPV, IPV, MMR, Hib, HBV)	
Contraindications	
Anaphylactic reactions to a vaccine contraindicate further doses to that vaccine. Anaphylactic reaction to a vaccine constituent contraindicates the use of vaccines containing that substance. Moderate or severe illnesses with or without a fever	Mild to moderate local reaction (soreness, redness, swelling) after a dose of an injectable antigen Mild acute illness with or without low-grade fever Current antimicrobial therapy Convalescent phase of illnesses Prematurity (use same dose and indications for normal, full-term infants) Recent exposure to an infectious disease History of penicillin or other nonspecific allergies or family history of such allergies
DTwP or DTaP	
Contraindications	
Encephalopathy within 7 days of administration of previous dose of DTP	Temperature $< 40.5°C$ (105°F) following a prior dose of DTP Family history of convulsions

True and False Contraindications and Precautions[17]	
True Contraindications and Precautions	**False (Vaccines May Be Administered)**
Precautions[a]	
Family history of Sudden Infant Death Syndrome Collapse or shock-like state (hypotonic-hyporesponsive episode) within 48 hours of receiving a prior dose of DTP Seizures within 3 days of receiving a prior dose of DTP Persistent, inconsolable crying lasting ≥ 3 hours within 48 hours of receiving a prior dose of DTP	Fever ≥ 40.5°C (105°F) within 48 hours after vaccination with a prior dose of DTP Family history of an adverse event following DTP administration
OPV	
Contraindications	
Infection with HIV or a household contact with HIV Known altered immunodeficiency (hematologic and solid tumors; congenital immunodeficiency; immunosuppressive therapy) Immunodeficient household contact	Breast-feeding Current antimicrobial therapy Diarrhea
Precaution[a]	
Pregnancy	
IPV	
Contraindication	
Anaphylactic reaction to neomycin or streptomycin	Infection with HIV
Precaution[a]	
Pregnancy	
MMR	
Contraindications	
Anaphylactic reaction to egg ingestion or to neomycin Pregnancy Known altered immunodeficiency (hematologic and solid tumors; congenital immunodeficiency; immunosuppressive therapy)	Tuberculosis or positive skin test Simultaneous tuberculin skin testing Pregnancy of recipient's mother Immunodeficient family member or household contact Infection with HIV
Precaution[a]	
Receipt of an immune globulin product within last 3 months	Nonanaphylactic reaction to egg or neomycin
Hib, Hepatitis B	
None identified	

[a] Events or conditions listed as precautions and not contraindications to immunization should be carefully reviewed, considering the benefits and risks of giving a specific vaccine to that individual.

Phase II: Decision-Making

By the beginning of the second phase, you will have gathered enough data to identify diseases to which the person is susceptible. Then you are ready to suggest a set of immunizations to protect the person against potential infections. The goal is to inform the person of immunization needs and convince him or her to receive these vaccines, considering the risks and benefits involved.[6]

In developing an immunization plan, consider age, occupation, place of residence, travel plans, lifestyle, underlying disease states and other individual factors. In consultation with detailed immunization reference books, construct a specific list and schedule of needed vaccines.

How to Read a Childhood Vaccine Schedule

To start, make sure you have a copy of the current childhood immunization schedule; look for a specific date. During the 1970s and early 1980s, the national immunization schedule hardly changed at all. Since 1985, it has been unusual for a year to go by without one or more major policy changes. Question any schedule that does not have a date on it.

The current national childhood immunization schedule can be obtained by contacting one of the following sources:

- Your local or state health department
- A recent issue of the *Morbidity & Mortality Weekly Report (MMWR),* either in print at a local library or via the Internet: http://www.cdc.gov/epo/mmwr/mmwr.html
- Via the Centers for Disease Control & Prevention's Internet web site: http://www.cdc.gov/ or http://www.cdc.gov/nip/whatnw.htm/.

Next, consider a specific child. Start with the top line and consider that disease and vaccine fully. Decide this child's vaccine needs for that line. Repeat for each successive line. Make sure to read all pertinent footnotes.

Note that bars on the childhood immunization schedule indicate ranges of acceptable ages for the corresponding vaccine. The "2-month" column applies to children as young as 6 weeks of age. This schedule represents a standard, most desirable schedule. To "catch-up" against a disease threat, intervals may be compressed or condensed to hasten immunity. Nonetheless, observe the minimum intervals discussed below.

Consult detailed references such as *ImmunoFacts* for information about storage, handling, dosage and administration unique to each vaccine or antibody.[4]

Call your county health department for availability of immunization records. Encourage patients and parents to take shot records to every health visit, and encourage full compliance with the national schedule. For children who missed the recommended vaccines at a certain age, schedule make-up visits as soon as possible.

Determining Adolescent and Adult Vaccine Needs

A checklist for adolescent immunization is provided here for your use. Use it in "catch-up" immunization programs. Several new vaccines were not available or not in use when today's teenagers were infants. Hepatitis B and varicella vaccines are the most obvious examples along with a second dose of measles-mumps-rubella (MMR) vaccine.[19]

For adults, the major concern is delivering influenza and pneumococcal vaccine. A table of vaccine issues for adults is provided. In addition to influenza and pneumococcal vaccines, MMR, varicella, hepatitis B and tetanus-diphtheria (Td) are described.

Timing of Adult Immunizations			
Measles-Mumps-Rubella (MMR)	One dose is recommended for adults born in 1957 or later if that person was not previously immunized. (A second dose may be required in some work or school settings.)		
Varicella	Two doses at least 30 days apart are recommended for anyone ≥ 13 years old with a negative history of varicella (chickenpox) or herpes zoster ("shingles").		
Hepatitis B for those at risk *	first dose	second dose 1 month later	third dose 5 months after second dose
Tetanus-Diphtheria (Td) if initial series not given during childhood	first dose	second dose 1 month later	third dose 6 months after second dose
If basic series complete	One dose every 10 years		

Timing of Immunizations For Older Adults and Those With Chronic Illnesses	
Influenza (flu)	Given yearly in the fall to people ≥ 65 years of age. Also recommended for people < 65 who have medical problems such as heart disease, lung disease, diabetes and other conditions and for others who work or live with high-risk individuals.*
Pneumonia	Given at ≥ 65 years of age. A repeat dose 6 years later may be given to those at highest risk.* Also recommended for people < 65 years of age who have kidney disorders, sickle cell anemia and chronic illnesses such as those listed for influenza.

Adolescent Immunization Checklist[19]

Make sure your clients from 11 to 21 years of age can document immunity or immunization against these diseases:

Recommended Immunizations	
Disease	Doses of Vaccine
Measles-Mumps-Rubella (MMR)	2 doses of vaccine
Varicella	Oral history of disease is adequate in this case, otherwise vaccinate. For those < 12 years old, give a single dose. For those ≥ 13 years old, give 2 doses of vaccine at least 1 to 2 months apart.)
Hepatitis B	3 doses of vaccine
Tetanus-Diphtheria Toxoids (Td)	0.5 ml dose every 10 years

Recommended Immunizations	
Disease	Doses of Vaccine
Influenza vaccine	For those with heart or lung disease or diabetes.
Pneumococcal vaccine	
For specific needs: Hepatitis A vaccine	Dosing schedule depends on age
Vaccines for international travel Other immunizations based on individual circumstances	Follow specific dosing requirements

* Consult your doctor, pharmacist or nurse to determine your level of risk.

Adapted from the Immunization Action Coalition, St. Paul, MN 55104.

TIMING AND SPACING OF VACCINES

Spacing Doses of the Same Vaccine

Increasing the interval between doses of a vaccine series does not diminish the effectiveness of a vaccine, but it does delay protection. Resume the recommended schedule as soon as possible. Additional doses are not needed, but if the patient has no records, vaccinate. Except for BCG, there is no such thing as overdosing on a vaccine. Vaccinating an immune person is not harmful.[20]

Decreasing the interval between doses of a vaccine to periods less than those recommended may interfere with overall immune response and protection.

In most cases, do not give doses of the same vaccine less than 4 weeks apart. For OPV, the minimum interval is 6 weeks between doses. For Hib vaccines, the minimum intervals vary; see detailed texts. Typically, you should wait 6 months between the penultimate (next-to-last) and ultimate doses of a series. An exception is Hib vaccine.

Do not count doses given inside the minimum interval. Wait the appropriate amount of time after the most recent dose and then give the next dose.

Timing in Relation to Antibodies

Inactivated vaccines generally do not interact with antibodies. Inactivated vaccines may be given at any time before or after giving antibodies.[20]

The immune response to live vaccines can be significantly impaired if given too close to a dose of antibody products or certain blood products. This is especially true for measles and varicella vaccines. Vaccinate 2 weeks before or wait 3 to 11 months after administering antibodies, depending on the antibody dose given.[21]

After IGIM, TIG and HBIG, wait 3 months before giving a live vaccine. After RIG, wait 4 months. After packed red blood cells, whole blood or high-dose IGIM, wait 6 months. After plasma, platelets or IGIV, wait 7 to 11 months. If a shorter interval is used, revaccinate after the appropriate interval or check the patient's antibody concentration and revaccinate if warranted.

General Rule: Adverse Events

The primary adverse events produced by live, attenuated vaccines mimic a mild case of the natural illness. They are most likely to occur after the incubation period of the natural infection. Inactivated vaccines are most likely to produce localized reactions at the injection site, with or without fever. Other adverse events may occur, but these general rules are the best way to summarize what to expect.[4,20]

General Rule: Contraindications and Precautions

A contraindication to vaccination is a condition in a recipient likely to result in a life-threatening problem if the vaccine is given. The standard contraindication for any vaccine is a severe allergic reaction (eg, immediate and life-threatening anaphylaxis) to a vaccine component after an earlier dose of that vaccine. This contraindication is not transferable. If someone develops anaphylaxis after receiving tetanus toxoid, it is reasonable to later give MMR.[4,20]

A precaution is defined as a condition in a recipient that may result in a life-threatening problem if the vaccine is given, or it could be a condition that may compromise vaccine efficacy. In these cases, weigh the risks and benefits for vaccine candidates individually. Precautions can often be considered as temporary or relative contraindications. Examples include:

- Pregnancy (for live vaccines, theoretically)
- Immunosuppression (live vaccines)
- Moderate to severe illness (address the acute need, then vaccinate)
- Recent receipt of a blood product (live vaccines)
- Immunosuppression
- Congenital immunodeficiency
- Leukemia, lymphoma, generalized malignancy
- HIV infection (contraindicates some live vaccines)
- Chemotherapy (alkylating agents, antimetabolites)
- Radiation therapy
- Corticosteroids: Prolonged therapy > 20 mg/d or > 2 mg/kg/d. Does not apply to topical steroids, inhaled steroids, alternate-day therapy or short-course (< 2 weeks) therapy.
- For more information, see chapter five on "Special Situations," or ACIP's statement on immunization of people with altered immunity.[22]

Phase III: Education and Consent

We have an immunization plan for this person; we need to explain it and gain the vaccinee's cooperation.[11] Sociologists recognize five key factors in a person's decision whether or not to be vaccinated:[1-3]

- Perceived susceptibility to a disease
- Perceived seriousness of a disease
- Perceived vaccine barriers (eg, side effects, access)
- Perceived vaccine benefits
- Social influence (like that of a pharmacist, nurse or physician)

Use these five issues and your knowledge of this person's particular situation to persuade him or her that immunization is worthwhile.

To convince someone of the importance of his or her immunization plan, language is crucial. Inform the person while avoiding medical jargon and confusing terms. Stop periodically to confirm that the person understands the conversation. Keep the tone and inflection of your voice positive and reassuring. Allow people to respond to your advice. Encouraging questions is important at this stage. Show empathy to convey acceptance and understanding. The dialogue below exemplifies a situation where a good introductory question sets the stage for teaching.

Motivator: Did you know that diabetes puts you at increased risk for some infections? Most of all, you are at high risk for influenza and pneumococcal infections. The good news is that effective vaccines can prevent these infections.

Vaccine Candidate: No, I wasn't aware that I was at risk or that vaccines are available. Can you tell me more?

An equally important part of counseling is nonverbal communication. Much can be learned from nonverbal cues, including the person's emotional state, level of understanding and need for further information. Maintain eye contact while talking. Preferably, the counselor is at the same eye level as the vaccine candidate. Watch facial expression to assess the individual's interest. Hesitation, a questioning glance, or any action out of the ordinary by the person can alert you to reevaluate the situation. Try not to read questions during the counseling session. Acknowledge the person's comments by nodding when appropriate. A relaxed posture will lessen the anxiety of the person and facilitate communication.

Make the environment for the counseling session quiet and private to reduce interruptions. Adequate lighting is important so nonverbal communication, lip reading and visual aids, are recognized. Avoid obstacles to communication, both physical and psychological barriers. Physical barriers include high counters, glass partitions and elevated platforms.

Using dedicated counseling rooms or a place away from congested areas can provide a private atmosphere that increases listening and learning. An obvious example of the need for confidentiality occurs with hepatitis B vaccine. Because many of the indications for this vaccine involve sexuality, it is important to cultivate a respectful relationship.

Give immunization advice verbally if it is simple. Written recommendations may be better if the person must follow a more complex schedule. It is helpful if you are prepared to explain specifically when and where to obtain immunization and what costs to expect. Providing written handouts can remind people of important points after they leave. Handouts are available from the CDC, state and local health departments, vaccine manufacturers and many other sources.[6,13,23-25]

The Power of Suggestion

You can put the power of suggestion to work with vaccines. If someone asks you for a dose of influenza vaccine, ask "Would you like pneumococcal vaccine as well?" This shows how astute you are, knowing that the indications for the two vaccines overlap among the elderly and people with some chronic illnesses.

If someone asks for a tetanus booster, you can respond "You need protection against diphtheria too. Let's make it combined tetanus-diphtheria toxoids (Td)."

If a parent brings younger children along with school-aged children to receive shots, check to see if they can be vaccinated against anything. If siblings did not tag along, remind the parent that all children, especially preschoolers, need to be protected against preventable infections.

Maybe you can think of other examples where you can suggest additional protection. Once you start checking someone's immune status, check for all that person's needs. Check the whole family, or ask the parent to bring all the records to the next visit.

Informed-Consent Documents

It is imperative that you obtain informed consent from vaccine candidates before administering vaccines. This is important for several ethical reasons and is required by law in some cases.[26]

Immunization usually involves giving a foreign protein to an otherwise healthy person. While modern vaccines are highly effective and highly safe, rare adverse events of high consequence occur rarely. Because of the minutely small but real risk of adverse events after vaccination, getting informed consent reflects that person's (or a parent's) autonomy in choosing whether or not to be protected.

Obtaining the signature that reflects informed consent is itself part of the procedure in educating and counseling people and reduces misunderstandings that can lead to lawsuits. Documented informed consent is required by law for vaccines purchased with federal funds and is the standard of practice in many communities even for vaccine purchased privately. Check with health departments for local requirements.

While some practices use shorter consent forms, thorough and specific forms (like the CDC-endorsed forms) are more likely to be judged meaningful by a court. Each begins with the phrase "What you need to know before you or your child gets vaccinated...." Vaccine information sheets for common vaccines are available from the CDC in several languages, including Armenian, Cambodian, Chinese, English, Farsi, Hmong, Japanese, Korean, Laotian, Portugese, Romanian, Russian, Samoan, Spanish, Tagalog and Vietnamese. French counterparts are available from Canadian authorities.

During the informed-consent process, explain honestly the benefits and risks of immunization to the person being vaccinated. Do this before the immunization is given. An informed-consent form should be signed by the person and the healthcare provider and kept on file. Professionals can help assure that the frequency and consequences of vaccine side effects are substantially less than the consequences of the disease to be prevented.

In obtaining informed consent for children, ensure that the consenting adult is authorized to provide consent. Specific cases will vary from state to state. Make sure that the consenting adult reads and understands the risk and benefits of the vaccine to be administered. Use the current recommended version of the consent form for each vaccine. Provide the consenting adult with a copy of the consent form with the clinic or practice telephone number stamped or attached to it. That number is important so adverse events after immunization can be reported or so questions can be answered. In the case of illiteracy or marginal literacy, read the consent form to the person.

Phase IV: Confirmation

The final part of the counseling process is the evaluation phase. By asking the person to summarize the material communicated, the counselor can determine if he or she comprehended the ideas discussed. An example of a person being counseled about immunizations for international travel is provided below.[6]

Motivator: We have talked about many things. Can you summarize which immunizations you need and other recommendations we covered?

Vaccine Candidate: I need vaccines against yellow fever and typhoid, which I can get from the health department on Main Street. I should be careful to eat and drink only certain foods and beverages during my trip. I should also take malaria tablets and use mosquito protection.

The ultimate success of immunization counseling is determined by whether or not the person is actually immunized. Immunization is favored if convenience is enhanced. Ask for the promise of a parent to obtain a child's immunizations by a certain date, and ask the person to report to you how he or she found the vaccination experience to be. Remind the person that the small inconvenience in being immunized is an investment in health that pays dividends for years to come. Suggest that they encourage friends with similar vaccine needs to be vaccinated as well.

Opportunities

The skills of interviewing and counseling to increase vaccine acceptance are not perfected overnight. Use lessons learned from talking with some people to help other individuals. You might want to research the immunization needs of your own family as a first step. Interviewing, asking relevant questions and screening high-risk people through medication use and medical history are also important. The process can provide people with information about their personal immunization needs.

Reminder and Recall Systems

Reminding parents of immunization visits improves appointment keeping. Recalling children who miss immunization visits decreases immunization drop-out rates. Both measures increase immunization coverage.

What is a reminder/recall system? The reminder part involves sending a timely mail or making a telephone call to notify parents of children due for upcoming vaccination visits. The recall portion involves a mail or telephone message to parents of children who missed a vaccination visit or are past due for a vaccination.

Reminder/recall systems can be manually operated or automated. Aggressively implemented, reminder/recall systems improve appointment compliance and vaccination coverage levels. Reminder/recall messages can be delivered by computer-generated mailings or telephone calls. Telephone numbers of the children to be reminded or recalled from form information or a computerized database of immunization records and telephone numbers can be linked to an "autodialer." Automated telephone dialers can average 80 to 100 completed messages per hour (over 25,000/month). They can contact people during evenings and weekends, redial busy and no-answer numbers and record messages from clients (eg, an appointment change).

For a manual recall system, enter each child into the recall system whenever the first immunization is administered. Record the vaccine on a suitable card, tell the parent when to return for the next dose, tab the card across the top corresponding to the month the child should return, then refile the card in the active file.

If a child returns on time, repeat the procedure outlined. If a child does not return on time, a reminder postcard is mailed to the parent. Send two reminder cards at least 1 month apart. If time and resources permit, telephone follow-up is effective.

Over the past 20 years, studies of manual telephonic or mailed appointment reminders showed significant improvements in compliance for a variety of scheduled health visits. A large case-control trial of autodialer-delivered immunization reminder/recall messages showed a 45% higher rate of immunization visits among message recipients (41%) compared with those not contacted (28%). In another study, a single call the night before the scheduled immunization visit improved visit compliance by 183%.

All reminder/recall systems require up-to-date client telephone numbers or addresses. The labor to maintain your database is essential to the effectiveness of these communication systems. If you adopt a reminder/recall system, use it aggressively. Send reminders before every scheduled appointment. Send recall messages immediately after any missed visit.

The cost-effectiveness of various reminder/recall systems varies according to practice size, degree of automation and other individual practice factors. In large- to medium-size practices, automated telephone dialers markedly reduce the operating costs incurred by manual reminder/recall systems and can pay for themselves through savings in postage costs. Automated technology is most cost-effective when computerized immunization records are available. In that case, after initial installation, little human intervention is required. Automated dialing technology is effective in offices and clinics using manually maintained records as telephone numbers can be entered quickly by hand into an "autodialer."

The CDC recommends that all public and private immunization providers use a reminder/recall system. Automated reminder/recall technology is simple, effective and inexpensive. For more information, contact the Program Operations Branch at the CDC's National Immunization Program, 404-639-8209.

References

[1] Riddiough MA, Willems JS, Sanders CR, et al. Factors affecting the use of vaccines: Considerations for immunization program planners. *Public Health Rep* 1981;96:528-35.
[2] Carter WB, Beach LR, Inui TS, et al. Developing and testing a decision model for predicting influenza vaccination compliance. *Health Service Research* 1986;20:897-932.
[3] Montano DE. Predicting and understanding influenza vaccination behavior: Alternatives to the health-belief model. *Med Care* 1986;24:438-53.
[4] Grabenstein JD. *ImmunoFacts: Vaccines & Immunologic Drugs.* St. Louis: Facts and Comparisons, Inc., May 1997.
[5] Grabenstein JD, Hayton B. Pharmacoepidemiologic program for identifying of patients in need of vaccination. *Am J Hosp Pharm* 1990;47:1774-80.
[6] Kirk JK, Grabenstein JD. Interviewing & counseling patients about immunizations. *Hosp Pharm* 1991;26:1006-10.
[7] Falvo DR. Communicating health advice. In: Raphael MG, Higgins ME, ed. *Effective Patient Education* Rockville, MD: Aspen Systems Corporation, 1985:127-55.
[8] Rosenstock IM. Why people chose health services. *Milbank Memorial Fund Quarterly* 1966;44:94-127.
[9] Svarstad BL. Physician-patient communication and patient conformity with medical advice. In: Mechanic D, ed. *The Growth of Bureaucratic Medicine: An Inquiry Into the Dynamics of Patient Behavior and the Organization of Medical Care.* New York: John Wiley & Sons, 1976:220-38.
[10] Janz NK, Becker MH. The health belief model: A decade later. *Health Educ Quarterly* 1984;11(Spring):1-47.
[11] Morris LA. *Communicating Therapeutic Risks.* New York: Springer Verlag, 1990.
[12] Rudd CC. Teaching and counseling patients about drugs. In: Ray MD, ed. *Basic Skills in Clinical Pharmacy Practice.* Carrboro, NC: American Society of Hospital Pharmacists, 1983:156-82.
[13] Tindall WN, Beardsley RS, Kimberlin CL. *Communication Skills in Pharmacy Practice,* 2nd ed. Philadelphia: Lea & Febiger, 1989:85-97.
[14] Brink SG. Provider reminders: Changing information format to increase infant immunizations. *Med Care* 1989;27:648-53.
[15] Margolis KL, Nichol KL, Poland GA, et al. Frequency of adverse reactions to influenza vaccine in the elderly: A randomized, placebo-controlled trial. *JAMA* 1990;264:1139-41.
[16] Klein N, Morgan K, Wansbrough-Jones MH. Parent's beliefs about vaccination: The continuing propagation of false contraindications. *Brit Med J* 1989;298:1687.
[17] Centers for Disease Control & Prevention. Standards for pediatric immunization practices. *MMWR* 1993;42(RR-5):1-13.
[18] Centers for Disease Control & Prevention. Recommended childhood immunization schedule-US, 1997. *MMWR* 1997;46:35-40.
[19] Advisory Committee on Immunization Practices. Immunization of adolescents. *MMWR* 1996;45(RR-13):1-16.
[20] Advisory Committee on Immunization Practices. General recommendations on immunization. *MMWR* 1994;43(RR-1):1-38.
[21] American Academy of Pediatrics. Recommended timing of routine measles immunization for children who have recently received immune globulin preparations. *Pediatrics* 1994;93:682-5.
[22] Advisory Committee on Immunization Practices. Recommendations of the Advisory Committee on Immunization Practices: Use of vaccines and immune globulins in persons with altered immunocompetence. *MMWR* 1993;42(RR-4):1-18.
[23] Ley P. *Communicating With Patients: Improving Communication, Satisfaction and Compliance.* New York: Croom Helm, 1988.
[24] Klein-Schwartz W, Hoopes JM. Patient assessment and consultation. In: Feldmann EG, Blockstein WL, Young LL, ed. *Handbook of Nonprescription Drugs,* 9th ed. Washington, DC: American Pharmaceutical Association, 1990:11-23.
[25] Morrow D, Leirer V, Sheikh J. Adherence and medication instructions: Review and recommendations. *J Am Geriatric Soc* 1988;36:1147-60.
[26] Fulginiti VA. Patient education for immunizations. *Pediatrics* 1984;74(S):961-3.
[27] American College of Physicians. *Guide for Adult Immunization,* 3rd ed. Philadelphia: American College of Physicians, 1994.
[28] Peter G, ed. *1994 Red Book: Report of the Committee on Infectious Diseases,* 23rd ed. Elk Grove Village, IL: American Academy of Pediatrics, 1994.

CHAPTER 5

Special Situations

Customizing Immunization Plans

Immunization policies are written to bring the greatest advantage in disease prevention to the most people. Even so, use of vaccines and antibodies must be tailored to each person.

This section reviews major groups of precautions and special situations that require individualized attention. The topics considered in turn include pregnancy, lactation, issues of advancing age, underlying disease and weakened immune systems.

Pregnancy

About 6% to 10% of clinically recognized pregnancies result in spontaneous miscarriage. Some 23% of conceptions result in other forms of preclinical embryo loss. Recognizable congenital malformations occur in about 3% to 5% of live births. Chance occurrence of any of these events after vaccination or use of any drug does not imply that the drug caused the event. Some adverse events occur randomly.[1]

The FDA's Pregnancy Categories are based on availability of information to rule out a drug risk to the fetus balanced against the drug's potential benefits to the mother. For most vaccines, human studies do not exist and animal studies are lacking. This is FDA's Pregnancy Category C. Risk cannot be ruled out, but potential benefits of the drug often justify the risk. This is the most common category, more for lack of data than for any evidence of danger.[2-9]

It is often appropriate to vaccinate a pregnant woman despite the designation Pregnancy Risk Category C. No licensed vaccine has ever been shown to cause birth defects, including attenuated rubella vaccine. On the contrary, vaccination may be of great value to the mother and the child. IgG antibodies begin crossing the placenta during the first trimester of pregnancy, but most is transferred during the third trimester. Neonatal serum IgG levels correlate with gestational age. Other immunoglobulin isotypes (eg, IgA, IgM) do not cross the placenta.[10]

Do not discharge a woman from a hospital or birthing center unless she is immune to rubella. Vaccinate susceptible women shortly after delivery, using measles-mumps-rubella (MMR) vaccine.

Note that about 4000 deaths from hemolytic disease of the newborn (HDN) still occur each year in the US. HDN results when an Rh-antigen negative woman develops anti-Rh antibodies and then has a later pregnancy with an Rh-antigen positive fetus. The mismatch between fetal antigens and maternal antibodies results in major birth defects and often fetal death. About 1500 of these deaths would be preventable if Rh_o(D) immune globulin were used more to prevent $Rh_o(D)$ isoimmunization. $Rh_o(D)IG$ should be used more following abortion, antepartum hemorrhage or amniocentesis. Be sure all women in need get $Rh_o(D)$ immune globulin to prevent isoimmunization.[11]

Recommendations for Immunization During Pregnancy	
Live Virus Vaccines	
Measles	Contraindicated (hazard is theoretical, not proven)
Mumps	Contraindicated (hazard is theoretical, not proven)
Rubella	Contraindicated (hazard is theoretical, not proven; in a study of > 700 vaccinated pregnant women, no fetal abnormalities were seen)
Varicella	Contraindicated (hazard is theoretical, not proven)
Yellow Fever	Contraindicated, unless exposure to yellow-fever virus is unavoidable.
Poliovirus	OPV is preferred when immediate protection is needed. Human studies have shown no hazard. IPV is an option if vaccination series can be completed before exposure.
Live Bacterial Vaccines	
BCG	Avoid use.
Typhoid (capsules)	Consider risk of disease and benefits of vaccine.
Inactivated Virus Vaccines	
Hepatitis B	Pregnancy is not a contraindication.
Influenza A & B	Recommended for patients with serious underlying disease. Consult each year's guidelines.
Hepatitis A	Use in people at high risk.
Poliovirus	OPV is preferred when immediate protection is needed. Human studies have shown no hazard. IPV is an option if vaccination series can be completed before exposure.
Rabies	Use in people with substantial risk of exposure.
Inactivated Bacterial Vaccines	
Pneumococcal	Use in people at high risk.
H. influenzae b	Use in people at high risk.
Meningococcal	Use in unusual outbreak situations.
Typhoid (injections)	Consider risk of disease and benefits of vaccine.
Toxoids	
Tetanus-diphtheria (Td)	Vaccinate if a woman lacks a primary series or if no booster was given within the past 10 years.
Immune Globulins	
Pooled or hyperimmune globulins	Use for exposure or anticipated unavoidable exposure to measles, hepatitis A, hepatitis B, rabies or tetanus.

Breast-Feeding

Breast-feeding is not a specific contraindication to immunization. Rubella vaccine-strain virus is secreted in milk and may be transmitted to infants in this manner. In infants infected with rubella this way, none exhibited severe disease. However, one exhibited mild clinical illness typical of acquired rubella. Even so, CDC recommends that breast-feeding not serve as a contraindication to infant or maternal immunization.[2-3,12-15]

Various nutritional, immunologic and other advantages of breast-feeding are known. Secretory IgA is the prevalent immunoglobulin in human milk, while IgG predominates in bovine milk. Secretory IgA protects infants against *Escherichia coli, Shigella, Salmonella, Campylobacter, Haemophilus influenzae, Streptococcus pneumoniae, Klebsiella pneumoniae,* polioviruses, rotaviruses, respiratory syncytial virus, influenza virus, cytomegalovirus and numerous other microbes. Secretory IgA antibodies are found in the feces of breast-fed infants by the second day of life, while only 30% of formula-fed infants had IgA in the feces by 1 month of age. IgM and IgG also may be present in breast milk, although in smaller concentrations than IgA. Maternal IgA is especially important until infants produce their own IgA at 4 to 12 months of age.

Issues of Age

Response to immunologic drugs may be slightly or significantly impaired with advancing age. Unfortunately, risk of death from influenza or pneumococcal disease increases with advancing age. For this reason, give pneumococcal vaccine as risk increases but before the immune response is impaired too greatly. This implies that people should be vaccinated promptly at age 65, even if they are healthy, rather than wait until their health is less robust at 70 or 75. Impaired responses to hepatitis B vaccine are seen in people above 40 years of age.[2-3,16]

ACIP and other authorities recommend a routine vaccination status assessment at age 50. Reviewing adult vaccination status, administering Td and determining whether the person has risk factors for pneumococcal and influenza vaccines are of special interest. Among adults 50 to 64 years of age with cardiovascular or pulmonary risk factors, only 9% to 15% of them had received pneumococcal vaccine. Only 21% to 28% had received influenza vaccine.[16,17-19]

Children < 2 years of age do not respond as well to polysaccharide vaccines as they do to protein antigens. Protein-based vaccines work well from infancy through adulthood.[11]

International Travel

There is insufficient space in this book to provide all information needed to operate a consultation service for immunizations and health advice for international travel. Several references provide counseling for the traveler and detailed vaccine requirement information by country. *ImmunoFacts: Vaccines & Immunologic Drugs* lists vaccines available abroad by generic and proprietary names plus immunologic terms in several languages.[5,11,20]

Underlying Disease

Use caution when giving any vaccine to someone with severely compromised cardiopulmonary status or in whom a febrile or systemic reaction could pose a significant risk. Any serious active infection is reason for delaying a vaccine except when withholding the vaccine entails a greater risk. Generally, do not administer immunologic drugs to someone with an unexplained fever until the cause of the fever is determined and evaluated. If the fever is caused by an infection, withhold the immunologic drug until the patient is afebrile unless the risk of withholding the drug outweighs the risk of immunization.[2-3]

In many cases, underlying disease is the clue or the trigger that prompts us to vaccinate someone. This is certainly true for influenza and pneumococcal vaccines where chronic cardiovascular, lung, metabolic, kidney or other diseases are the actual indication for vaccination. Do not forget to immunize hospitalized children.[2-3,21-28]

People with chronic liver disease should be vaccinated against hepatitis A and hepatitis B. With hepatitis B, kidney dialysis, hemophilia, thalassemia, panacinar emphysema (using of alpha$_1$-proteinase inhibitor) and repeated sexually transmitted diseases are indications for immunization.

A table of diseases that are indications for vaccination is provided in the chapter two on "Too Many Deaths, Too Much Disease." Adjacent to that table is a table of the medications that help identify the people with those diseases. These lists are useful for searching automated medical records or prescription databases to find people at elevated risk.

To find these people, harness all the administrative tools at your disposal. Use your quality-assurance or quality-improvement program. Collaborate with your utilization review and discharge planning staffs.

Use critical pathways developed in your institution involving congestive heart failure, diabetes, asthma, pneumonia, dialysis, splenectomy, chemotherapy, radiation therapy and the like. Take advantage of critical pathways for post-myocardial infarctions, stroke, orthopedics and those involving any organ. Everyone needs to have his or her immunization status updated periodically. Try to make up missed immunization opportunities for children, adolescents or adults at your practice site.

Develop standing orders for the emergency department, pediatrics, labor and delivery, dialysis, transplant and coronary care units, diabetic clinics and the like.

WEAKENED IMMUNE SYSTEMS

Two concerns affect immunization recommendations for people with weakened immune systems. The first is the immune response that can be expected when these individuals are immunized. The second concern is the types of immunizations needed directly because of reduced resistance to natural infection.[2-3,28-30]

Immunodeficiency: Immune Response

People with immune deficiencies may not respond sufficiently to immunizing agents. They may remain susceptible to infection despite appropriate vaccination. Immunization is frequently recommended for them with the hope that they gain at least partial immunity. Firm advice on impairment degree of the immune response and solid data on proper timing of vaccine doses in relation to immunosuppressive drug or radiation therapy are unavailable. Some rules are discussed below.[2-3,29-31]

If the immunocompromise is temporary, consider deferring immunization until several months after immunosuppressive treatment is discontinued. If feasible, measure specific serum antibody concentrations or other immunologic responses at an appropriate interval after immunization. Consider risk-benefit ratios for individual patients and consult current authoritative guidelines.

Inactivated Products: Giving inactivated vaccines to people with impaired immune responses is not dangerous; these immunizations may not yield the expected antibody response. This may occur whether the immunocompromise is caused by the use of immunosuppressive therapy (eg, irradiation, antimetabolites, alkylating agents, cytotoxic agents, large doses of corticosteroids), a genetic defect, HIV infection, leukemia, lymphoma, generalized malignancy or other causes. Short-term corticosteroid therapy (< 2 weeks) or intra-articular, bursal or tendon injections of corticosteroids are usually not immunosuppressive nor is topical, aerosol or replacement therapy.

Live, Attenuated Products: Immunization with live bacterial or viral organisms in immunocompromised patients is generally contraindicated because of the risk of vaccine-induced infection. This may occur with immunosuppressive therapy (eg, irradiation, antimetabolites, alkylating agents, cytotoxic agents, large doses of corticosteroids), a genetic defect, HIV infection, leukemia, lymphoma, generalized malignancy or other causes. Short-term corticosteroid therapy (< 2 weeks) or intraarticular, bursal or tendon injections of corticosteroids are usually not immunosuppressive nor is topical, aerosol or replacement therapy. Steroid doses > 2 mg/kg or > 20 mg/day is likely to suppress immune responses.

Without definite data to base timing decisions, a common rule is to vaccinate people ≥ 2 weeks before immunosuppressive therapy to allow time for an antibody response. Alternately, wait > 3 months after stopping high-dose steroids or other immunosuppressive therapy for best efficacy. Longer waits in organ transplant recipients are common.

Never give live oral poliovirus vaccine (OPV) to immunocompromised people or members of their family, rather use the parenteral inactivated poliovirus vaccine (IPV). Measles-mumps-rubella (MMR) vaccination is recommended for asymptomatic children infected with HIV. Also consider it for symptomatic HIV-positive children. MMR vaccination in such children has not been associated with serious or unusual adverse effects, but antibody responses have been variable.

Antibodies: The therapeutic value of immune globulins is not impaired in immunocompromised people. Individuals with selective immunoglobulin A deficiency may develop anti-IgA antibodies and could have anaphylactoid reactions to subsequent administration of blood products (including immune globulin preparations) that contain IgA.

Immunodiagnostic Skin Tests: Immunocompromised people may have a diminished skin-test response to immediate- and delayed-hypersensitivity antigens. Skin-test responsiveness also may be suppressed by active tuberculosis and other bacterial or viral infection, malnutrition, malignancy or immunosuppression.

Immunodeficiency: Infection Risk

Immunosuppression increases the risk of infection and the need for vaccine protection. Oncology patients, organ transplant recipients, people without functioning spleens and people with other primary or acquired forms of immunodeficiency are especially vulnerable. The cancer concern especially applies to people with leukemia, lymphoma, a generalized malignancy and those receiving chemotherapy or radiation therapy. Asplenia might be anatomic (eg, after trauma) or functional (eg, from sickle-cell disease). Other causes of immune compromise include renal failure or nephrotic syndrome, diabetes mellitus (types I and II) and alcoholism or alcoholic liver disease.[2-3,29-31]

The infectious threats to these individuals start with the usual microbes that would menace them if they did not have an immune deficiency. To this list, influenza and pneumococcal disease can be added in most cases. Further, people with Hodgkin's disease, people without functioning spleens and people with HIV infection are at greater risk than normal of infection with capsular bacteria. Vaccinate them with *Haemophilus influenzae* type b (Hib) and meningococcal A/C/Y/W-135 vaccines. For Hib vaccine, give adults a single 0.5 ml dose of any brand.

Some of these people may need hepatitis B vaccine. As mentioned earlier, live vaccines are generally avoided in immunosuppressed people. An exception is varicella vaccine where a special protocol is available for children with acute lymphoblastic leukemia (ALL).

Timing of immunizations is usually challenging. The best option is to vaccinate 2 to 4 weeks before the immune system is suppressed. Organ transplant candidates can be vaccinated while on organ waiting lists. If advance prophylaxis is not possible, vaccinate during disease remission > 3 months after chemotherapy or radiation therapy.

Because of the seasonal threat of influenza, it may not be feasible to wait that many months before the threat arrives. Some sources recommend waiting just 3 to 4 weeks after therapy, so long as peripheral granulocytes and lymphocytes exceed 1000 cells/mm^3. The fact that this is an inactivated vaccine aids this decision.

Vaccinate asplenic people ≥ 2 weeks before elective splenectomy, or they can be vaccinated after acute recovery from their splenectomy.

Policies vary among transplantation centers, but inactivated vaccines are often deferred for 1 to 2 years and MMR vaccine for 2 years after transplantation. Do not give live vaccines to anyone with chronic graft-vs-host disease (GVHD).

VACCINES FOR PEOPLE INFECTED WITH HIV

Live Bacterial or Viral Vaccines

Special immunization recommendations are appropriate for people infected with HIV.[2-3,11,30,32-34]

People infected with HIV and people with AIDS are theoretically at risk of disseminated infection if they are immunized with a live, albeit attenuated, vaccine. Specific recommendations follow:

BCG (injection or instillation): Disseminated mycobacterial infection may result from exposure to this drug. Do not expose HIV-infected people in the US to BCG. BCG vaccination of children who are born to HIV-infected mothers in developing nations and who are vaccinated shortly after birth appear to be relatively safe but questionably effective. WHO recommends that only HIV-infected infants who are asymptomatic and live in areas with high tuberculosis risk receive BCG.

Measles, mumps and rubella (MMR): Vaccinate both symptomatic and asymptomatic children and adults according to routine schedules. Less than optimal immune responses may result.

Poliovirus (oral form, OPV): Do not administer live, oral poliovirus vaccine to any HIV-infected child or adult in the US nor to their household contacts. Do give inactivated poliovirus vaccine (IPV) injection. WHO continues to recommend routine use of OPV as a rational approach in developing nations with a substantial risk of endemic poliomyelitis.

Typhoid (capsule form): Do not administer live, oral typhoid vaccine to any HIV-infected child or adult. Inactivated typhoid vaccine injection may be used if needed.

Vaccinia (smallpox): Do not administer live vaccinia (smallpox) vaccine to any HIV-infected child or adult.

Varicella (chickenpox): Do not administer live varicella vaccine to any HIV-infected child or adult, until further information is published. Consider the value of VZIG for immunocompromised people.

Yellow fever: Base decisions to administer live yellow-fever vaccine to an HIV-infected individual on extent of immunosuppression and the risk of exposure to the yellow-fever virus. Offer the option of immunization to asymptomatic people infected with HIV who cannot avoid potential exposure to yellow-fever virus.

Inactivated Vaccines or Toxoids

In general, immunization with an inactivated vaccine or toxoid poses no additional risk to HIV-infected people and AIDS victims. These individuals may be less likely to develop an adequate immune response to vaccination and may remain susceptible to disease. While HIV-infected people and AIDS patients may develop less than optimal immunity compared with uninfected people immunization is often still recommended to confer at least partial protection. Complete immunization of HIV-infected people before they meet the criteria for AIDS. Specific recommendations follow; keep in mind that less than optimal immune responses may result with any of these vaccines.

Cholera: Use standard recommendations. Encourage food and water precautions.

Diphtheria & tetanus toxoids with pertussis vaccine (DTP): Use routine pediatric DTP vaccination schedules for HIV-infected children.

Diphtheria & tetanus toxoids (pediatric): Use routine pediatric DT vaccination schedules for HIV-infected children. DTP is the preferred drug for almost all children.

***Haemophilus influenzae* type b (Hib):** Use routine pediatric Hib vaccination schedules for HIV-infected children. Routine Hib vaccination of all HIV-infected adolescents and adults is generally recommended to decrease susceptibility to Hib disease. Complete immunization of HIV-infected people before they meet the criteria for AIDS.

Hepatitis A: Use standard recommendations.

Hepatitis B: Use routine pediatric hepatitis B vaccination schedules for HIV-infected children. Routine hepatitis B vaccination of all HIV-infected adults (unless already infected with hepatitis B) is generally recommended to decrease susceptibility to hepatitis B infections. Complete immunization of HIV-infected people before they meet the criteria for AIDS.

Influenza: Routine influenza vaccination of all HIV-infected people is generally recommended to decrease susceptibility to influenza infections. Chemical antiviral prophylaxis (eg, rimantadine) may be appropriate during periods of increased influenza activity in a community.

Meningococcal A/C/Y/W-135: Use standard recommendations.

Plague: Use standard recommendations.

Pneumococcal: Routine pneumococcal vaccination of all HIV-infected people is generally recommended to decrease susceptibility to pneumococcal infections. Complete immunization of HIV-infected people before they meet the criteria for AIDS.

Poliovirus (injection, IPV): Use standard recommendations. IPV is preferred over the oral, attenuated poliovirus vaccine.

Rabies: Use standard recommendations.

Tetanus & diphtheria (Td adult): Routine Td vaccination of all HIV-infected adults is recommended to decrease susceptibility to tetanus and diphtheria infections. Research suggests a lower threshold for using TIG in wounded HIV-infected people under the assumption that circulating antitetanus antitoxin may be lower than among uninfected people.[35]

Typhoid (injection): Use standard recommendations. Encourage food and water precautions.

Safety of Immunizing HIV-Infected People

In vitro studies show that proliferating CD4 cells are more susceptible to infection with HIV than nonproliferating cells. This raises the possibility that immunization may be a cofactor in the progression of HIV infection to AIDS. Recent reports show temporary increases in plasma HIV viremia after injection of tetanus toxoid or influenza or hepatitis B vaccines. These increases lasted up to 6 weeks. Clinical data have not shown that antigenic stimulation leads to deterioration of clinical status. We encounter natural antigenic stimulation innumerable times during our lives. Actual infections may be riskier than an immunization because of more prolonged antigenic stimulus. The risk to an HIV-infected person from a vaccine is probably outweighed by the value of induction of specific antibodies. CDC and WHO continue to recommend immunization of HIV-infected people as described above, when the benefits of immunization outweigh the risks.[30,36-39]

Summary Recommendations for Routine Immunization of HIV-Infected People in the US

Drug	Known Asymptomatic	Symptomatic
DTP/Td	yes	yes
OPV	no	no
IPV[a]	yes	yes
MMR	yes	yes[b]
Hib[c]	yes	yes
Pneumococcal	yes	yes
Influenza	yes[b]	yes
Varicella[d]	no	no

[a] for adults > 18 years of age, use only if indicated
[b] consider risk and benefit
[c] consider for HIV-infected adults
[d] awaiting results of clinical studies in HIV-infected children

References

[1] Cunningham FG, MacDonald PC, Leveno KJ, et al. *Williams Obstet rics,* 19th ed. Norwalk, CT: Appleton & Lange, 1993:661-90,919-38.
[2] Advisory Committee on Immunization Practices. Update on adult immunization: Recommendations of the Immunization Practices Advisory Committee. *MMWR* 1991;40(RR-12):1-94.
[3] American College of Physicians. *Guide for Adult Immunization,* 3rd ed. Philadelphia: American College of Physicians, 1994.
[4] Barry M, Bia F. Pregnancy and travel. *JAMA* 1989;261:728-31.
[5] Centers for Disease Control & Prevention. *Health Information for International Travel.* Washington, DC: Government Printing Office, revised annually and updated biweekly.
[6] Halsey NA, Klein D. Maternal immunization. *Pediatr Infect Dis J* 1990;9:574-81.
[7] Harjulehto-Mervaala T, Aro T, Hiilesmaa VK, et al. Oral polio vaccination during pregnancy: Lack of impact on fetal development and perinatal outcome. *Clin Infect Dis* 1994;18:414-20.
[8] Insel RA. Maternal immunization to prevent neonatal infections. *N Engl J Med* 1988;319:1219-20.
[9] Ornoy A, Ben Ishai P. Congenital anomalies after oral poliovirus vaccination during pregnancy. *Lancet* 1993;341:1162.
[10] American College of Obstetricians & Gynecologists. Technical Bulletin #160: Immunization during pregnancy. Washington, DC: ACOG, October 1991.
[11] Grabenstein JD. *ImmunoFacts: Vaccines & Immunologic Drugs.* St. Louis: Facts and Comparisons, Inc., May 1997.
[12] Slade HB, Schwartz SA. Mucosal immunity: The immunology of breast milk. *J Allergy Clin Immunol* 1987;80:346-56.
[13] Goldman AS. The immune system of human milk: Antimicrobial, anti-inflammatory and immunomodulating properties. *Pediatr Infect Dis J* 1993;12:664-72.
[14] Losonsky GA, Fishaut JM, Strussenberg J, et al. Effect of immunization against rubella on lactation products. I. Development and characterization of specific immunologic reactivity in breast milk. *J Infect Dis* 1982;145:654-60.
[15] Losonsky GA, Fishaut JM, Strussenberg J, et al. Effect of immunization against rubella on lactation products. II. Maternal-neonatal interactions. *J Infect Dis* 1982;145:661-6.
[16] Centers for Disease Control & Prevention. Assessing adult vaccination status at age 50 years. *MMWR* 1995;44:561-3.
[17] Centers for Disease Control & Prevention. Influenza and pneumococcal vaccination coverage levels among persons aged ≥ 65 years – US, 1973-1993. *MMWR* 1995;44:506-7,513-5.
[18] Centers for Disease Control & Prevention. Pneumonia and influenza death rates – US, 1979-1994. *MMWR* 1995;44:535-7.
[19] Centers for Disease Control & Prevention. Mortality patterns – US, 1993. *MMWR* 1996;45:161-4.
[20] World Health Organization. *International Travel & Health: Vaccination Requirements & Health Advice.* Albany, NY: WHO, revised annually.
[21] Fulginiti VA. Incomplete immunizations, hospitalization, and specialty care: An opportunity to improve the immunization status of very young children. *Am J Dis Child* 1988;142:704.
[22] Tifft CJ, Lederman HM. Immunization status of hospitalized preschool-age children: The need for hospital-based immunization programs. *Am J Dis Child* 1988;142:719-20.
[23] Riley DJ, Mughal MZ, Roland J. Immunisation state of young children admitted to hospital and effectiveness of a ward-based opportunistic immunisation policy. *Brit Med J* 1991;302:31-3.
[24] Fedson DS, Baldwin JA. Previous hospital care as a risk factor for pneumonia: Implications for immunization with pneumococcal vaccine. *JAMA* 1982;248:1989-95.
[25] Grabenstein JD, Hayton BD. Pharmacoepidemiologic program for identifying patients in need of vaccination. *Am J Hosp Pharm* 1990;47:1774-81.
[26] Fedson DS, Harward MP, Reid RA, et al. Hospital-based pneumococcal immunization: Epidemiologic rationale from the Shenandoah study. *JAMA* 1990;264:1117-22.
[27] Ruben FL. Who needs influenza vaccine? In: Kendal AP, Patriarca PA, ed. *Options for the Control of Influenza.* New York: Alan R. Liss, Inc., 1986:139-54.
[28] US Preventive Services Task Force. *Guide to Clinical Preventive Services,* 2nd ed. Baltimore: Williams & Wilkins, 1996.
[29] Hibberd PL, Rubin RH. Approach to immunization in the immunosuppressed host. *Infect Dis Clin N Amer* 1990;4:123-42.

[30] Advisory Committee on Immunization Practices. Recommendations of the Advisory Committee on Immunization Practices: Use of vaccines and immune globulins in persons with altered immunocompetence. *MMWR* 1993;42(RR-4):1-18.

[31] Kafidi KT, Rotschafer JC. Bacterial vaccines for splenectomized patients. *Drug Intell Clin Pharm* 1988;22:192-7.

[32] Onorato IM, Markowitz LE, Oxtoby MJ. Childhood immunization, vaccine-preventable diseases and infection with human immunodeficiency virus. *Pediatr Infect Dis J* 1988;7:588-95.

[33] Steinhart R, Reingold AL, Taylor F, et al. Invasive Haemophilus influenzae infections in men with HIV infection. *JAMA* 1992;268:3350-2.

[34] Peter G, ed. *1994 Red Book: Report of the Committee on Infectious Diseases,* 23rd ed. Elk Grove Village, IL: American Academy of Pediatrics, 1994.

[35] Furste W. The potential development of tetanus in wounded patients with AIDS: Tetanus toxoid and tetanus immune globulin. *Arch Surg* 1986;121:367.

[36] Steinhoff MC, Auerbach BS, Nelson KE, et al. Antibody responses to *Haemophilus influenzae* type b vaccines in men with human immunodeficiency virus infection. *N Engl J Med* 1991;325:1837-42.

[37] Pau AK, McNicholl IR, Pursell KJ. Active immunization with HIV-infected patients. *Pharmacotherapy* 1996;16:163-70.

[38] Stanley SK, Ostrowski MA, Justement JS, et al. Effect of immunization with a common recall antigen on viral expression in patients infected with human immunodeficiency virus type 1. *N Engl J Med* 1996;334:1222-30.

[39] Glesby MJ, Hoover DR, Farzadegan H, et al. The effect of influenza vaccination on human immunodeficiency virus type 1 load: A randomized, double-blind, placebo-controlled study. *J Infect Dis* 1996;174:1332-6.

CHAPTER 6

Immunization Administration

General Issues

This chapter begins with consensus recommendations on proper injection technique.[1-9] Even if you are experienced, never give an injection with an attitude of indifference or routine. Attention to detail and sound knowledge of the anatomy involved is essential. Understand the terms that describe the injection site precisely. Injecting a medication incorrectly can cause nerve injury and pain, bleeding or a sterile abscess.

Preparation and caution are essential to injections. Injections introduce two foreign objects into the body, a needle and the medication. Precision of dosing and movement are key. A misdirected injection may prevent medication from acting as intended or may cause damage.

Wash your hands and the preparation area. Assemble the necessary supplies.

Prepare the Patient

Wearing gloves usually is not recommended during an injection, but check local recommendations. Wear gloves if you will come into contact with potentially infectious body fluids or have open lesions on your hands. Discard gloves and put on new gloves before seeing the next person. Observe universal precautions to avoid contact with body fluid. Wash hands between patients.

Expose a wide area to permit an unobstructed view of the injection site. Rotate among usable sites when repeated injections are necessary.

Wipe the intended injection site with an appropriate antiseptic agent (eg, soap and water, povidone-iodine, 70% isopropyl alcohol). Start at the center of the intended injection site and move outward. Optimally, wait 5 minutes before injection to allow the germicide to work. Most caregivers wait for alcohol to evaporate before proceeding.

Few children are completely cooperative. Because they may struggle when least expected, take steps to calm the child during the injection. Restraining an uncooperative client may require two people.

Prepare the Dose

Visually inspect any parenteral drug for particulate matter and discoloration before administration when solution and container permit. If particulate matter or abnormal discoloration are noted, discard that container and submit appropriate drug quality reports.

Remove protective covers from the vials you will use. Treat the stoppers of parenteral drug containers with an appropriate disinfectant (eg, 70% isopropyl alcohol). Optimally, allow the disinfectant to work 5 minutes before opening or piercing the container with a needle. Most caregivers wait for alcohol to evaporate before proceeding.

Use the recommended diluent for each powdered drug to avoid physical or chemical incompatibility and inactivation of the drug. Reconstitute live vaccines with diluents that do not contain antimicrobial preservatives (eg, phenol, thimerosal). Use the specific quantity required to obtain the proper concentration.

Gently agitate suspensions before withdrawing each dose to disperse the contents and obtain a uniform suspension. Do not shake protein solutions vigorously, because foaming can lead to protein denaturation. Gentle rotation or swirling will achieve thorough mixing.

Draw a volume of air into a sterile syringe equal to the volume of liquid drug to be withdrawn. Next, pierce the center of the rubber stopper in the vial, invert the vial, and slowly inject the air in the syringe into the vial. Keeping the tip of the needle immersed, withdraw the desired volume of liquid drug; or use a negative-pressure method by retracting the plunger to withdraw the product and then allowing air in the syringe to flow into the vial to offset the vacuum created. Then, holding the syringe plunger steady, withdraw the needle from the vial.

Double-check vial labels and volume measurements for accuracy. Be sure you have the correct person, drug, dose, route and timing. Handle materials aseptically.

Deliver the Dose

Promptly inject the drug to avoid settling of the suspension in the syringe. After inserting the needle, pull back on the plunger to check for entry into a vessel. If blood appears in the needle hub, withdraw the needle and select a new site. Discard the contents of that first syringe. Repeat this process at a different injection site until no blood appears, then push down on the plunger. After injecting the fluid, withdraw the needle in one smooth motion along the same angle as insertion. Apply pressure to site with cotton swab to discourage bleeding. Apply an adhesive bandage if needed. For multiple doses, use different extremities or sites.

Use a separate needle and syringe for each person to avoid transmission of hepatitis B and other blood-borne infectious agents. Use disposable needles and syringes only once. Sterilize reusable glass syringes and needles by autoclaving at 121°C (250°F) for 30 minutes or use appropriate dry heat; alcohol is not effective. Hepatitis B has been transmitted via common-source contamination of multidose vials and jet injectors.[10-12]

Discard used needles and syringes without recapping into a rigid, puncture-resistant container, often called a sharps container. Dispose of these containers according to local hazardous waste procedures. If you are not part of a larger institution, you may need to hire a contractor to haul away these containers. Such contractors are often found in the telephone book. Consider any specific state regulations regarding biohazard disposal.

If the drug product includes no preservative, discard unused portions of the container after a single use. The most commonly used preservatives in parenteral drugs are thimerosal, phenol, benzyl alcohol and parabens (eg, methylparabens, propylparabens). Document the procedure.

CHOOSING A ROUTE

Subcutaneous (SC) injections are usually absorbed more slowly than intramuscular (IM) injections. It may slightly reduce the antibody concentrations ultimately obtained if a vaccine intended for IM administration is given SC. If an *IM* vaccine is inadvertently given *SC,* do not give the patient another dose. The antibody response from the inadvertent SC injection will not be as strong as what would be obtained IM, but the difference is not enough to warrant another vaccine dose.

SC fat in the gluteal area may interfere with responses to an adsorbed vaccine. Give adults and children adsorbed vaccines in the deltoid area, usually IM. Avoid injection into the gluteus maximus because of the potential for sciatic nerve damage, especially in infants.

Intramuscular Injection

Vaccines given IM include diphtheria-tetanus-pertussis (DTP) vaccines, diphtheria-tetanus toxoids for pediatric use (DT), tetanus-diphtheria toxoids for adult use (Td), influenza, *Haemophilus influenzae* type b (Hib), hepatitis B, and pneumococcal vaccines. Do not use gluteal muscles except for immune globulin intramuscular (IGIM). If the gluteal region is used, avoid the central region. Use only the upper, outer quadrant. Avoid major peripheral nerve trunks.[13]

Generally, vaccines containing an adjuvant are injected IM. SC or intradermal (ID) injection of these vaccines may cause local irritation, induration, skin discoloration, inflammation or granuloma formation. Preferred IM injection sites are the anterolateral aspect of the upper thigh muscle, for young children, and the deltoid muscle of the upper arm.

Select a target muscle large enough to accommodate the volume to be injected. Deposit medication into the belly of the muscle for optimal absorption. A relaxed muscle is desirable. A slow rate of injection allows the relaxed muscle to distend and accommodate the fluid injected. Too rapid a rate of injection into a taut muscle can result in expulsion of the medication from the muscle into surrounding tissues, causing severe irritation and discomfort. Select a needle long enough to reach the muscle mass and prevent vaccine from seeping into SC tissue but not so long that it endangers underlying neurovascular structures or bone. Base needle size and site of injection on the person's age, volume of drug, size of the muscle and the depth below the muscle surface into which the drug is to be injected.

For infants < 12 months of age, the thickest point of the anterolateral aspect of the thigh muscle provides the largest muscle mass, the vastus lateralis. Use the greater trochanter and the knee as landmarks. Look for a suitable site two fingers' breadth below the trochanter and two fingers' breadth above the knee in the outer aspect of the thigh. This should point to the middle third of this muscle. Do not inject into the medial thigh, where major blood vessels and nerves are found. Usually, a ⅝- to 1-inch, 22- to 25-gauge needle will penetrate the thigh muscle of a 4-month-old infant.

The deltoid muscle also can be used, such as when multiple vaccines are administered during the same visit. The deltoid muscle in infants and young children is shallow and can accommodate only a small volume of the more fluid medications. Another limiting factor is that repeated injections in this area are painful.

When the anterolateral surface of the upper thigh is used, the needle is directed distally (toward the knee) and inserted at a 90° angle to the horizontal and long axes of the leg. The needle should not penetrate deeper than 1 inch. Compressing the muscle tissues between the fingers amasses the musculature at the site of injection.

For toddlers and older children, needle size for the deltoid can range from 22 to 25 gauge and from ⅝ to 1¼ inches. For the anterolateral thigh, use a longer needle, ⅞ to 1¼ inches.

For adults, the thickest point of the deltoid muscle is preferred with a needle size of 20 to 25 gauge and 1 to 1½ inches. One method is to place four fingers across the deltoid muscle with the top finger along the acromion process. Look for a suitable injection site three fingers' breadth below the acromion process. Another method is to make a "C" with the thumb and forefinger. When the forefinger is on the acromion process, look for an injection site in the center of the "C." Flexing the arm at the elbow or relaxing the deltoid muscle will allow a more comfortable injection.

Analysis of deltoid fat pad thickness in adults suggests the following needle selections: for men, 1- to 1½-inch needles; for women < 70 kg (154 lbs), use a 1-inch needle; for women > 70 kg, use a 1½-inch needle; for women > 100 kg (220 lbs) and obese men, consider a 2-inch needle. Many pre-filled syringes have a ⅝-inch needle attached. These shorter needles appear to be acceptable for lean, slender people.

Guide to Intramuscular Injection

Group	Site	Needle Length	Gauge
Infants	thigh	⅝-1″	22-25
Older children	deltoid	⅝-1¼″	22-25
	thigh	⅞-1¼″	22-25
Adult men	deltoid	1-1½″	20-25
Women < 70 kg (154 lbs)	deltoid	1″	20-25
Women 70 to 100 kg	deltoid	1½″	20-25
Women > 100 kg (220 lbs) and obese men	deltoid	consider 2″	20-25

Tap the syringe to remove any liquid on the needle. Pull the protective cover off the needle. With one hand, stretch the skin taut around the injection site. Hold the syringe horizontally with the other hand until ready for injection. Warn the person that you are about to inject. Insert the needle into the muscle with a quick thrust at a 90° angle. Expect to feel some resistance.

Once inserted, release the stretched skin and gently pull back slightly on the plunger and check for blood. If there is blood in the syringe, do not use it. Get a new set of materials and begin again. If you do not see blood, slowly push the plunger until the syringe is empty. See the following table for further details.

Hold a cotton ball near the needle at the injection site and pull the needle straight out using the same angle as entry. Use the cotton ball to apply pressure to the site for a few seconds or rub gently in a circular motion. If there is bleeding at the site, wipe it off and, if necessary, apply an adhesive bandage. Dispose of supplies properly, including the diluent.

A site often chosen for its ease of access is the deltoid area. It can be used when the recipient is in a standing, sitting or prone position. While the deltoid muscle forms a fairly large triangle on the shoulder prominence, the area available for a shoulder injection is limited because there are major bones, blood vessels and nerves to be avoided. The recommended injection area is a rectangle bounded by the lower edge of the acromion on the top and lateral side of the arm opposite the axilla or armpit on the bottom. The two side boundaries are lines parallel to the arm ⅓ and ⅔ of the way around the outer lateral aspect of the arm. Avoid the acromion, clavicle, humerus, the brachial veins and arteries and the radial nerve. Limit the number and size of injections at this site. The area is small and cannot tolerate repeated injections and large volumes.

Give IM injections with caution to persons on anticoagulant therapy or with bleeding tendencies. IM hepatitis B immunization of 153 hemophiliacs with a 23-gauge needle, followed by steady pressure (without rubbing) to the injection site for 1 to 2 minutes, resulted in a 4% bruising rate with no patients requiring factor supplementation.[14-15]

Subcutaneous Injection

Vaccines given SC are deposited beneath skin and fat but above muscle. SC vaccines include the various combinations of measles, mumps and rubella vaccines, inactivated poliovirus vaccine (IPV), pneumococcal vaccine and varicella vaccine and allergen-extract immunotherapy. If an *SC* vaccine is inadvertently given *IM,* do not repeat the dose. Antibody response after inadvertent SC injection will be less than IM, but the difference is not enough to warrant another vaccine dose.[13]

SC injections are intended for tissue below the dermal layer of the skin, either the outer aspect of upper arm or the fatty area of the anterolateral thigh. SC injections are usually administered into the thigh of infants or the deltoid area of older children and adults.

Use a ⅝- to ¾-inch, 23- to 25-gauge needle to inject into the tissues below the dermal layer of the skin. Pull the protective cover off the needle. With one hand, pinch up ≈ 1″ of SC tissue to help prevent inadvertent IM administration. The needle should be ≈ ½ as long as the skinfold is wide.

Guide to Subcutaneous Injection		
Group	Needle Length	Gauge
Infants	⅝-¾″	23-25
Children and adults	⅝-¾″	23-25

Hold the syringe with the other hand until ready for injection. Warn the recipient that you are about to inject. Then insert the needle at a 45° angle into SC tissue with the bevel facing upward using a smooth motion.

Once inserted, release the skin and gently pull back slightly on the plunger and check for blood. If there is blood in the syringe, do not use it. Get a new set of materials and begin again. If you do not see blood, slowly push the plunger until the syringe is empty.

Hold a swab or wipe near the needle at the injection site and pull the needle straight out using the same angle as entry. Use the wipe to apply pressure to the site for a few seconds or rub gently in a circular motion. If there is bleeding at the site, wipe it off and, if necessary, apply an adhesive bandage. Dispose of all supplies properly, including the diluent.

Intradermal Injection

Several immunologic drugs are given intradermally (ID). These include purified protein derivative (PPD) of tuberculin, some pre-exposure rabies vaccinations, some typhoid booster doses and some allergen skin tests.[13]

ID injections are commonly administered on the volar (ventral) surface of the forearm. Find an appropriate injection site one hand's breadth below the antecubital space and one hand's breadth above the wrist. The site should not be scarred, inflamed or covered with hair follicles. Otherwise, skin reactions will be hard to evaluate. Use a ⅜- to ⅝- inch, 25- to 27-guage, short-bevel needle. This is the Mantoux technique. ID reactions after pre-exposure human-diploid cell rabies vaccination are less severe when given in the deltoid area.

Stretch the skin with pressure of the opposite thumb. With the bevel facing upward, insert the needle into the epidermis at an angle parallel to the long axis of the forearm. Insert the needle at a 5° to 15° angle, so the entire bevel penetrates the skin. The needle tip should be visible through the skin. Properly injected solution will raise a small bleb or bubble, ≈ 0.5 cm in diameter.

Do not give an ID injection SC. This may result in a suboptimal immunologic response. Hepatitis B vaccine, for example, is effective ID at a lower dose than IM. The Centers for Disease Control and Prevention does not recommend its use in this way, because improper technique could leave vaccinees vulnerable.[16]

Do not massage the injection site.

Oral Administration

Only a few vaccines are administered orally. The most common one is live, attenuated oral poliovirus vaccine (OPV). One way to prevent typhoid fever is an oral capsule vaccine. Oral adenovirus vaccine tablets are used in some military basic training settings. Oral cholera vaccines are licensed in Europe and may soon be in the US. At least one of these involves initially swallowing an oral bicarbonate buffer solution, followed several minutes later by the acid-unstable vaccine.[13]

OPV is stored frozen in plastic units. Remove each unit from the freezer just before use. Rub it between the palms to thaw. Its normal color is pink from the phenol red added as a pH indicator. Color variation from red to yellow is acceptable. Next, squirt its contents into the recipient's mouth. For children, push up on the chin or tap the cheeks to assure swallowing. If an infant regurgitates much of an OPV dose within 5 to 10 minutes, give another dose during the same visit. Otherwise, readminister that dose at the next visit. Treat the empty OPV container as biohazardous waste for disposal.

The regimen for typhoid vaccine capsules is one capsule every other day for a total of four doses. Swallow each capsule 1 hour before meals with water no warmer than body temperature. Refrigerate the capsules between doses throughout the course of 7 days.

Synthesis

Proper injection technique must be mastered by anyone intending to immunize. The important thing is to learn this technique and begin protecting patients from debilitating and often fatal infections. Fifty to eighty thousand Americans die each year because no one warned them of their vulnerability to infection and offered them protection.

Before your patients leave, reinforce the need for additional vaccine doses they may require. Make return appointments while parents or the patient is still there. Write down for them the date the next doses are due. If you wish, have the parent or patient self-address reminder postcards that you can mail later. If necessary, reschedule missed appointments promptly.

Your patients deserve your proactive attention to prevention.

Emergency Plans

Rarely, immunization leads to anaphylaxis. This risk is statistically remote, ≈ 1 in 100,000 to 1 million or more doses, but it is highly consequential to the person involved.

The standard of care in many places is to have epinephrine readily available (eg, *EpiPen* autoinjector) and personnel trained in basic cardiac life support/cardiopulmonary resuscitation (BCLS/CPR). CPR training is available from the American Red Cross and other sources. In addition, immunization sponsors should know how to call for further competent assistance.[17-19]

Develop your emergency response plan in detail and practice it before administering immunizations. Post the appropriate epinephrine doses based on weight and age near your injection area for ready reference. Have telephone numbers of nearby physicians, hospitals and emergency medical services posted at a site visible from the telephone.

Response to a Systemic Reaction

Anaphylactic shock can be the most dramatic medical condition. Fortunately, most anaphylaxis is not fatal. The most important thing to remember is that the person who is immediately available to the patient is going to determine the outcome.[17-19]

Rarely will all of the following measures be necessary. Promptness in beginning emergency treatment is of utmost importance. For this reason, keep patients under observation of a competent caregiver for 15 to 30 minutes after vaccinating. Allow adequate space where you immunize to allow for fainting without injury to the patient. Have emergency supplies available, such as a stethoscope and blood-pressure cuff (pediatric and adult sizes). Keep the staff's certifications in basic cardiac life support and cardiopulmonary resuscitation (BCLS/CPR) current.

Anaphylaxis begins with apprehension and flushing. The patient will likely have sudden onset of itching, redness, or swelling of the lips, face or throat, with or without hives. Generalized itching over large portions of the body indicates the development of a more severe systemic reaction. Other possible symptoms include sneezing or coughing. Bronchospasm or shock may develop, with tightness or pain in the chest. Wheezing and shortness of breath, hoarseness and respiratory stridor may be present. This may lead to cyanosis, pallor and a weak or absent pulse.

All this occurs within minutes after an injection. If itching and swelling are confined to the extremity where the injection was given, observe the patient closely for 30 minutes, then refer for medical evaluation.

If symptoms extend beyond that extremity, place the patient in a supine position on a hard surface, elevating the feet if possible. Have someone call an ambulance or a physician immediately. Establish an oral airway, if necessary. Apply a tourniquet above the injection site, and inject 0.3 to 0.5 ml of epinephrine 1:1000 SC or IM into another extremity. Either the anterior thigh or deltoid muscle will suffice. SC is appropriate for mild or early cases. Use an IM injection for severe cases.

Monitor the patient's vital signs closely until assistance arrives. If the pulse disappears, administer CPR until the patient responds or the ambulance arrives. Maintain airway as needed. If oxygen is available, consider administering it by nasal cannula at 2 to 4 L/min.

The epinephrine dose may need to be repeated at 15- to 20-minute intervals, more frequently in severe cases. A succession of small doses is more effective and less dangerous than a single large dose. Loosen the tourniquet at least every 10 minutes.

The proper dose of SC epinephrine 1:1000 based on weight is:

kg	lbs	dose
3-15	6-33	0.1 mg/0.1 ml
16-25	34-55	0.2 mg/0.2 ml
26-35	56-77	0.3 mg/0.3 ml
36-45	78-99	0.4 mg/0.4 ml
≥ 46	≥ 100	0.5 mg/0.5 ml

The approximate dose of SC epinephrine 1:1000 based on standard body weights for age follows:

age	dose
2 to 6 months	0.07mg/0.07ml
12 months	0.1mg/0.1ml
1½ to 4 years	0.15mg/0.15ml
5 years	0.2mg/0.2ml
6 to 9 years	0.3mg/0.3ml
10 to 13 years	0.4mg/0.4ml
≥ 14 years	0.5mg/0.5ml

Repeat this dose every 5 to 20 minutes, based on individual response. Summon additional help if needed, and refer the patient to an appropriate source of follow-up care. Observation for several hours may be appropriate. Biphasic and protracted anaphylaxis, 5 to > 24 hours later, has occurred despite adequate initial management.

In general, the pediatric dose is 10 mcg (0.01 ml of a 1:1000 w/v solution) per kg body weight or 300 mcg (0.3 ml)/m^2 of body surface, up to 500 mcg (0.5 ml). Note that the *EpiPen Jr.* products contain 1:2000 w/v, suitable for children < 30 kg (66 lbs).[13]

Failing to give epinephrine promptly is more dangerous than using it improperly. Dosing epinephrine based on body weight is preferred. Too much epinephrine can lead to palpitations, tachycardia, flushing or headache. These reactions are unpleasant but pose little danger.

After adequate epinephrine has been given and if symptoms of angioedema, urticaria, rhinitis or conjunctivitis do not respond rapidly, inject an antihistamine (eg, diphenhydramine, *Benadryl*) IV or IM, according to the manufacturer's directions. Subsequent therapy might require use of corticosteroids, beta-adrenergic agonists or other drugs.

The proper dose of diphenhydramine based on weight is 1 mg/kg (50 mg maximum). A dosing chart for oral, IM or IV administration follows:

kg	lbs	dose	age	dose
3-15	6-33	10 mg		
16-25	34-55	20 mg	0-24 months	10 mg
26-35	56-77	30 mg	2-8 years	20 mg
36-45	78-99	40 mg	≥ 9 years	30 mg
≥ 46	≥ 100	50 mg		

Patients receiving beta-adrenergic antagonists (eg, beta-blockers) may be refractory to the effects of epinephrine. They may need additional epinephrine doses. Further, difficulty in maintaining blood pressure and pulse may last hours longer than in uncomplicated anaphylactic treatment.

Other measures that may be necessary include inhaled or parenteral bronchodilators or oxygen for cyanosis; endotracheal intubation, tracheotomy, cricothyrotomy or transtracheal catheterization for laryngeal edema; resuscitation, defibrillation, IV sodium bicarbonate and other proper medication(s) for cardiac arrest; mechanical airway use if the patient becomes unconscious; and oral or IV corticosteroids if the reactions may be prolonged. Monitor hypotension, and, if necessary, give vasopressors with adequate plasma volume replacement.

Remind patients and parents to report adverse events.

Comparison of Epinephrine for Self-Injection

Epinephrine Comparisons, for Self Administration			
Proprietary Name	*Ana-Kit* (and similar kits)	*EpiPen* and *EpiE-ZPen*	*EpiPen Jr.* and *EpiE-ZPen Jr.*
Manufacturer	Bayer and others	Center	Center
Concentration	1:1000, 1 mg/ml	1:1000, 1 mg/ml	1:2000, 0.5 mg/ml
Packaging	Manual syringe	Auto-injector	Auto-injector
Number of epinephrine doses per device	2	1	1
Dose delivered	2 doses of 0.3 mg/ 0.3 ml or other combinations	1 dose of 0.3 mg/ 0.3 ml	1 dose of 0.15 mg/ 0.3 ml
Number of chlorpheniramine doses per device	Four tablets of 2 mg each	None	None
Needle	25-gauge, ⅝-inch	original: 23-gauge, ½-inch EZ: 22-gauge, ⅝-inch	original: 23-gauge, ½-inch EZ: 22-gauge, ½-inch
Other components	2 alcohol swabs, tourniquet, case with belt clip	EZ versions feature an easy trigger and a belt clip	

Other Urgent Situations

Most emergencies related to immunizations do not involve anaphylactic shock. More commonly, they are anxiety reactions, such as simple fainting. Occasionally, hyperventilation with consequent respiratory alkalosis is seen. Breath-holding, even to the point of unconsciousness also may be seen, especially in children. Remember that though these situations may be dramatic, they usually do not represent a life-threatening situation. Obviously, secondary injury resulting from a fall may produce serious medical problems. This section, adapted from guidelines of the Texas Department of Health, reviews other events where quick responses may be necessary.

Fainting

Many clinicians have experienced a patient fainting before a procedure. Another term for this is a vasovagal reaction. "Fainters" can sometimes be spotted by their unusually quiet behavior, little interest in the procedure, slight pallor of the face and slight perspiration. Fainting generally does not represent a serious threat to the patient, but secondary injury can result from falling.

Fainting is characterized by loss of consciousness, normal vital signs, pallor and slight perspiration. Patients may report dizziness or a sensation that the room is enclosing around them. Check pulse, respiration and blood pressure. Keep the patient supine and elevate the lower extremities. Check the patient for secondary injury. The patient must be seen by a physician if there is any question of injury. Ammonia smelling salts may be used to stimulate consciousness. Do not give anything orally. Allow the patient to sit or stand only after the patient has completely stabilized and then only with support.

Hyperventilation

Hyperventilation occurs when an anxious patient breathes too rapidly and lowers the level of carbon dioxide in the blood, producing symptoms of respiratory alkalosis. Hyperventilation is accompanied by the feeling of breathlessness and anxiety. There is no wheezing, but there are often complaints of tingling or numbness in the extremities, light-headedness or dizziness. Occasionally cramping of the hands and feet occur. Unconsciousness is also a potential consequence.

The most obvious symptom is rapid respiration. A large volume of air is moved, and the chest expands and contracts well. Respirations may be deeper than normal. Blood pressure is normal to slightly elevated. Pulse is normal to slightly elevated. The patient may lose consciousness.

To treat hyperventilation, give the patient firm reassurance. Convince the patient to hold his or her breath. Alternately, have the patient close one nostril, breathing through the other nostril with the mouth closed. Breathing into a paper bag is a poor choice.

Breath-Holding

A person can voluntarily hold his or her breath until it produces symptoms, sometimes leading to unconsciousness. Because this situation usually involves a child, and the cyanosis it produces is prominent, the tendency is to become alarmed. Breath-holding in itself is harmless. Even when carried to the extreme of unconsciousness, respiration resumes once the patient loses consciousness. The only precaution needed is guarding against secondary injury. A brief transient seizure may be seen after the episode.

If seen when the child is still conscious, respirations may be absent. Cyanosis increases with time, while the blood pressure is normal. Pulse is normal to slightly elevated, but it may decrease during the breath-holding phase. The patient may lose consciousness.

If the patient is still conscious, place him or her in supine position. Check blood pressure, pulse and respirations. No other specific therapy is necessary. If the patient is unconscious before being noticed, check blood pressure, pulse and respirations to make sure that a more serious situation does not exist. Breath-holders regain consciousness quickly. Check for secondary injury. Blowing air or splashing water in the face may interrupt the breath-holding episode. Usually just holding and reassuring the child is sufficient.

Seizures

The primary concern in attending a person having a seizure is to prevent self-injury and inhalation of vomit. Seizures or convulsions involve a state of involuntary spasm or muscle contraction with loss of consciousness.

Protect the patient from falling, hitting the head or striking arms or legs against a hard surface. Lay the patient on either side or, if this is not possible, turn the head to one side. Do not force the jaw open. Do not put your fingers or any object in the patient's mouth. If respirations cease for longer than ½ to 1 minute, initiate resuscitative measures.

Observe events before, during and after the seizure and document them in the patient's record. This information may prove helpful to the patient's physician in determining causation. Refer the patient promptly for medical evaluation.

Upper Respiratory Obstruction

The patient may use the universal distress signal: Clutching the neck between thumb and index finger. Patients with a respiratory obstruction will gasp for air, be unable to speak or cough, appear cyanotic and have a foreign object blocking the airway.

Administer the Heimlich maneuver or CPR as necessary. Call for an ambulance or a physician if needed. Refer patient to a physician for follow-up.

References

[1] Smith-Temple J, Johnson JY. *Nurses' Guide to Clinical Procedures,* 2nd ed. Philadelphia: JB Lippincott Co., 1994:632-61.

[2] Swearingen PL. *Photo Atlas of Nursing Procedures,* 2nd ed. Redwood City, CA: Addison-Wesley Nursing, 1991:95-110.

[3] Perry AG, Potter PA. *Clinical Nursing Skills & Techniques.* St. Louis: CV Mosby, 1994:540-69.

[4] Suddarth DS. *Lippincott Manual of Nursing Practice,* 5th ed. Philadelphia: JB Lippincott Co., 1991:1145-8.

[5] Craven RF, Hirnle CJ. *Fundamentals of Nursing: Human Health & Function,* 2nd ed. Philadelphia: JB Lippincott Co., 1996:600-28.

[6] Wyeth Laboratories. *Intramuscular Injections.* New York: 1977.

[7] Laboratory Centre for Disease Control. Adsorbed vaccine injection technique. *Can Dis Weekly Rep* 1985;11:32.

[8] Laboratory Centre for Disease Control. Clarification: Adsorbed vaccine injection technique. *Can Dis Weekly Rep* 1985;11:56.

[9] Laboratory Centre for Disease Control. Immunization injection techniques. *Can Dis Weekly Rep* 1986;12:115-6.

[10] Centers for Disease Control. Hepatitis B associated with jet gun injection – California. *MMWR* 1986;35:373-6.

[11] Oren I, Hershow MD, Ben-Porath E, et al. A common-source outbreak of fulminant hepatitis B in a hospital. *Ann Intern Med* 1989;110:691-8.

[12] Centers for Disease Control. Improper infection-control practices during employee vaccination programs – District of Columbia and Pennsylvania, 1993. *MMWR* 1993;42:969-71.

[13] Grabenstein JD. *ImmunoFacts: Vaccines & Immunologic Drugs.* St. Louis: Facts and Comparisons, May 1997.

[14] Evans DIK, Shaw A. Safety and intramuscular injection of hepatitis B vaccine in haemophiliacs. *Brit Med J* 1990;300:1694-5.

[15] Advisory Committee on Immunization Practices. General recommendations on immunization. *MMWR* 1994;43(RR-1):1-38.

[16] Centers for Disease Control. Inadequate immune response among public safety workers receiving intradermal vaccination against hepatitis B – United States, 1990-1991. *MMWR* 1991;40:569-72.

[17] Thibodeau JL. Office management of childhood vaccine-related anaphylaxis. *Can Fam Phys* 1994;40:1602-10.

[18] Peter G, ed. *1994 Red Book: Report of the Committee on Infectious Diseases,* 23rd ed. Elk Grove Village, IL: American Academy of Pediatrics, 1994:49-51.

[19] Health Canada. Anaphylaxis: Statement on initial management in nonhospital settings. *Can Comm Dis Rep* 1995;21:200-3.

Visit Sketches

For detailed information about these vaccines, refer to *ImmunoFacts: Vaccines & Immunologic Drugs.*

Birth	
Vaccine	Hepatitis B
Dose #	#1
Dose	Depends on brand
Route	IM
Site	Anterolateral thigh
Needle	22 to 25 gauge ⅝ to 1″
Key Questions	Is mother HBsAg+? If yes, child needs HBIG.

2 Months of Age				
Vaccine	Hepatitis B	DTaP	IPV *	Hib
Dose #	#2	#1	#1	#1
Dose	Depends on brand	0.5 ml	0.5 ml	0.5 ml
Route	IM	IM	SC	IM
Site	Anterolateral thigh	Antero-lateral thigh	Antero-lateral thigh	Anterolateral thigh
Needle	22 to 25 gauge	22 to 25 gauge	22 to 25 gauge	22 to 25 gauge
	⅝ to 1″	⅝ to 1″	⅝ to 1″	⅝ to 1″
Key Questions or Comments	Is mother HBsAg+? If yes, baby needs HBIG.	Consider acetaminophen.		

* IPV is recommended by CDC and ACIP. If OPV is to be given, ask if child or any household member is immunosuppressed. If not, give one unit orally.

4 Months of Age			
Vaccine	DTaP	IPV *	Hib
Dose #	#2	#2	#2
Dose	0.5 ml	0.5 ml	0.5 ml
Route	IM	SC	IM
Site	Anterolateral thigh	Anterolateral thigh	Anterolateral thigh
Needle	22 to 25 gauge	22 to 25 gauge	22 to 25 gauge
	⅝ to 1″	⅝ to 1″	⅝ to 1″
Key Questions or Comments	Any prior reactions? Consider acetaminophen.		

* IPV is recommended by CDC and ACIP. If OPV is to be given, ask if child or any household member is immunosuppressed. If not, give one unit orally.

6 Months of Age				
Vaccine	Hepatitis B	DTaP	OPV *	Hib
Dose #	#3	#3	#3 **	#3
Dose	Depends on brand.	0.5 ml	0.5 ml	0.5 ml
Route	IM	IM	Oral	IM
Site	Anterolateral thigh	Anterolateral thigh	Mouth	Antero-lateral thigh
Needle	22 to 25 gauge	22 to 25 gauge	22 to 25 gauge	22 to 25 gauge
	⅝ to 1″	⅝ to 1″	⅝ to 1″	⅝ to 1″
Key Questions or Comments	Is mother HBsAg+? If yes, baby needs HBIG.	Any prior reactions? Consider acetamin-ophen.		

* OPV is recommended by CDC and ACIP. Alternately, IPV can be used.

** Third dose of poliovirus vaccine, first dose of OPV. Can be given from 6 to 18 months of age.

12 to 18 Months of Age			
Vaccine	DTaP	OPV	Hib
Dose #	#4	#3 **	#4
Dose	0.5 ml	0.5 ml	0.5 ml
Route	IM	Oral	IM
Site	Anterolateral thigh	Mouth	Anterolateral thigh
Needle	22 to 25 gauge	n/a	22 to 25 gauge
	⅝ to 1″	n/a	⅝ to 1″
Key Questions or Comments	Any prior reactions? Consider acetaminophen.	Immunosuppressed? If yes, use IPV.	
Vaccine	MMR	Varicella	Hepatitis B
Dose #	#1	#1	***
Dose	0.5 ml	0.5 ml	Depends on brand.
Route	SC	SC	IM
Site	Outer, upper arm	Deltoid	Anterolateral thigh
Needle	22 to 25 gauge	22 to 25 gauge	22 to 25 gauge
	⅝ to 1″	⅝ to 1″	⅝ to 1″
Key Questions or Comments	Severe allergy to gelatin, neomycin or egg? If yes, use caution.	Immunosuppressed? If so, consider deferring.	

* Ask if child or any household member is immunosuppressed. If not, give one unit orally.
** Third dose of poliovirus vaccine, first dose of OPV. Can be given from 6 to 18 months of age.
*** Opportunity to vaccinate those who have not had disease and not previously been vaccinated.

4 to 6 Years of Age					
Vaccine	DTaP	OPV *	MMR	Varicella	Hepatitis B
Dose #	#5	#4 **	#2	***	***
Dose	0.5 ml	0.5 ml	0.5 ml	0.5 ml	Depends on brand.
Route	IM	Oral	SC	SC	IM
Site	Deltoid or anterolateral thigh	Mouth	Outer, upper arm	Deltoid or anterolateral thigh	Deltoid or anterolateral thigh
Needle	22 to 25 gauge	n/a	22 to 25 gauge	22 to 25 gauge	22 to 25 gauge
	⅝ to 1″	n/a	5.8/ to 1″	⅝ to 1″	⅝ to 1″
Key Questions or Comments	Any prior reactions?	Immunosuppressed? If yes, use IPV	Severe allergy to gelatin, neomycin, or egg? If yes, use caution.	Immunosuppressed? If so, consider deferring.	

* Ask if child or any household member is immunosuppressed. If not, give one unit orally.
** Fourth dose of poliovirus vaccine, second dose of OPV. Alternately, IPV may be used.
*** Opportunity to vaccinate those who have not had disease and not previously been vaccinated.

11 to 21 Years of Age				
Vaccine	Td	MMR	Varicella	Hepatitis B
Dose	0.5 ml	0.5 ml	0.5 ml	Depends on brand.
Route	IM	SC	SC	IM
Site	Deltoid	Outer, upper arm	Deltoid	Deltoid
Needle	20 to 25 gauge	20 to 25 gauge	20 to 25 gauge	20 to 25 gauge
	1 to 1½″	1 to 1½″	1 to 1½″	1 to 1½″
Key Questions or Comments	Any prior reactions?	Severe allergy to gelatin, neomycin, or egg? If yes, use caution.	Immuno-compromised? If so, consider deferring.	

Adults 21 to 64 Years of Age					
Vaccine	Td	MMR	Varicella	Influenza	Pneumo-coccal
Dose	0.5 ml	0.5 ml	0.5 ml	0.5 ml	0.5 ml
Route	IM	SC	SC	IM	IM or SC
Site	Deltoid	Outer, upper arm	Deltoid	Deltoid	Deltoid
Needle	20 to 25 gauge	20 to 25 gauge	20 to 25 gauge	20 to 25 gauge	20 to 25 gauge
	1 to 1½″	1 to 1½″	1 to 1½″	1 to 1½″	1 to 1½″
Key Questions or Comments	Any prior reactions?	Severe allergy to gelatin, neomycin, or egg? If yes, use caution.	Immunocom-promised? If so, consider deferring	Severe allergy to gelatin, neomycin, or egg? If yes, use caution. For those with heart or lung disease or diabetes.	For those with heart or lung disease or diabetes.

Adults ≥ 65 Years of Age			
Vaccine	Td	Influenza	Pneumococcal
Dose	0.5 ml	0.5 ml	0.5 ml
Route	IM	IM	IM or SC
Site	Deltoid	Deltoid	Deltoid
Needle	20 to 25 gauge	20 to 25 gauge	20 to 25 gauge
	1 to ½″	1 to ½″	1 to ½″
Key Questions or Comments	Any prior reactions?	Severe allergy to gelatin, neomycin, or egg? If yes, use caution.	

These tables are provided as a service. They may be freely reproduced for individual clients, if credit is given to: Grabenstein JD. *Immunization Delivery: A Complete Guide.* St. Louis: Facts and Comparisons, 1997:90.

CHAPTER 7

Immunization Documentation

Data about care and progress are needed by the health professionals from many disciplines and specialties who contribute to a person's care. Like records for other prescription drugs, accurate immunization records are essential to document protection, to establish the proper timing for "refills" (eg, booster doses) and to preclude unneeded immunization.[1,2]

Immunization data are needed by all health professionals who care about disease prevention. To guide decisions, information about a history of previous immunizations must be readily available. Usually, data are recorded in medical records, although pharmacy records increasingly reflect use of preventive medicines. Standardization of records improves the efficiency and accuracy of data retrieval.

Memory and Recall

Two hazards threaten the accuracy of immunization records: Forgetting actual immunizations and imagining nonexistent ones. The two hazards have different causes and different solutions.[1]

Forgetfulness is a characteristic of patients and healthcare professionals. An example is when one clinician is unaware that another clinician immunized a patient. Adults may be especially vulnerable to individual and collective forgetfulness and are likely to have complicated medical histories. Pieces of their medical records are often kept with multiple office-based physicians, plus hospitals and other sites where care has been provided. The adult-immunization movement is a relatively recent phenomenon. Many adults have not yet had the benefit of a comprehensive immunization-needs assessment. Centralization of immunization documents helps assure complete access to such data.[3-6]

Imaginary immunizations may be recorded if people are asked leading questions, such as "You've had all your vaccinations, haven't you?" Undocumented assertions of vaccination are unreliable. Unsubstantiated claims of previous infection or vaccination may come from susceptible persons and claims of susceptibility may come from immune persons. In one study, offspring were more likely to provide "I don't know" answers than their mothers; offspring and parents also may report histories differently. These possibilities reinforce the importance of having written immunization records available to other decision makers. The one notable exception is varicella: Studies have shown that oral histories of chickenpox or herpes zoster are reliable.

Only through accurate immunization records available to clinicians and patients can the shortcomings of memory and recall be solved. The following sections address specific forms and types of immunization records.

Vaccine Records for Clinicians

Clinicians can use five types of documents for proper proof of immunization: (1) Medical records, (2) pharmacy records, (3) forms for collecting immunization histories (screening forms), (4) informed-consent forms and (5) records of adverse events temporally associated with immunization.[1,7]

The following is a screening form you can refine for your practice. The key questions are annotated with comments for responding to the person's answers. An immunization-screening form is appropriate for:

- Assessing the immunization needs of clients of private physicians and public health clinics;
- Assessing the immunization needs of people admitted to a hospital or an emergency room or entering nursing homes, schools or other institutions;
- Assessing employees' immunization needs, helping immunization programs run by occupational-health personnel; and
- Screening people for vaccination during influenza seasons or outbreaks (eg, measles, pertussis). Although the form is intended to consider children and adults, it is not specifically designed for well-baby screening. Another more specific form may be appropriate in such cases.

Most significantly, this form allows *individual* assessment of a person's indications and contraindications for vaccination. Using this instrument can turn a mass vaccination program into many individualized immunization encounters. It serves as a summary of immunization history to date as well as a record of immunizations ordered and administered as a result of that day's work. Data about tuberculin skin tests also can be recorded.

Annotated Screening Form

Part I: To be completed by patient or family:

1.) Age: ____.

2.) Date of birth: ______. Recommend annual influenza and initial pneumococcal vaccination for everyone ≥ 65 years old, even if otherwise healthy. People born in 1957 or later need two MMR doses. Base other immunization decisions on tables detailed in chapter 6.

3.) What is your daytime telephone number? (____) ____-_________
Telephone numbers are useful for reminding people to return for the next dose of vaccine or to receive tuberculin skin test results.

4.) Have you ever had a *serious* reaction to any vaccine that required medical care? If yes, please describe. ______________________
Severe allergic reactions (immediate, anaphylactic, life-threatening ones) generally contraindicate further vaccinations with that or related products. For children, ask about problems within 7 days after earlier vaccinations: Fever ≥ 105°F, seizures, continuous crying for ≥ 3 hours, unusual sleepiness, unusual high-pitched scream, collapse or unresponsiveness. Other reactions are largely irrelevant. Be wary of inappropriate contraindications that do not exclude people who need to be vaccinated.

5.) Are you pregnant? (circle one) No Yes Maybe
If pregnant or planning pregnancy in the next 3 months, be cautious with live vaccines. Inactivated vaccines are generally safe in pregnancy and may be important to protect the woman's health. Consider deferring live vaccines until after delivery, counsel to avoid pregnancy or consider risk/benefit ratio.

6.) Do you have substantial fever, diarrhea, or vomiting today? (circle one) No Yes
If illness is sufficient to warrant hospitalization or referral to the next higher level of care, defer vaccination until the acute event stabilizes, then vaccinate promptly. Low-grade fever is not a contraindication to vaccination. Make notes on deferred immunizations, to remind them to resume their immunizations.

7.) Do you have drug or food allergies? (circle one)
No Yes egg gelatin other: ______
Describe reaction: ________________________________

   a.) If eggs or gelatin cause laryngeal swelling or other severe systemic reactions, use influenza, measles, mumps and yellow-fever vaccines cautiously.

   b.) For anaphylactic-type antibiotic allergy to streptomycin (eg, polio) or neomycin (eg, polio, measles, mumps, rubella), avoid related vaccine. No vaccine currently available in the US or Canada contains penicillin.

   c.) Hypersensitivity to tetanus antitoxin (containing equine serum) may be erroneously reported as allergy to tetanus toxoid; clarify circumstances, type and onset of reaction.

8.) Are you or is anyone in your home receiving chemotherapy or radiation therapy? Is there anyone with HIV infection, AIDS or any immune disorder in your home?
Do you or anyone in your house have any form of immunosuppression? (circle one) No Yes
If yes, be cautious with use of live vaccines. For example, IPV may be preferred over OPV in these settings.

9.) Has this person received blood or antibodies (immune globulins) in the past 3 to 11 months? (circle one) No Yes Maybe
If so, be cautious with live vaccines. Timing between antibodies and vaccination depends on the dose of antibody given.

10.) Have you ever had a *positive* tuberculosis (TB) test?
(circle one) No Yes
When? ______
If patient has a history of positive tuberculin skin test (TST), do not rechallenge with PPD or old tuberculin (OT). Do not give BCG vaccine.

11.) Are you being treated by a doctor for: (circle all that apply to you)
- a.) Cancer (type: _______): Recommend influenza and pneumococcal vaccines. Patients on chemotherapy may have a diminished response but still warrant immunization. Do not give these people live vaccines if immunosuppressed.
- b.) Seizures or other neurologic problems: Do not give pertussis vaccine to children with evolving neurologic disorders. Wait for condition to stabilize. See detailed references for full discussion.
- c.) Diabetes: Recommend influenza and pneumococcal vaccines.
- d.) Heart or vascular disease: For congestive heart failure, septal defect, ischemic heart disease, atherosclerosis, intermittent claudication, valvular problems, angina, myocardial infarction, aneurysms, dysrhythmias, stroke and related conditions, recommend influenza and pneumococcal vaccines.
- e.) Hodgkin's disease: Recommend influenza and pneumococcal vaccines 2 weeks before or 1 to 3 months after radiation or chemotherapy.
- f.) Immunosuppression from drugs, radiation, etc.: Recommend influenza and pneumococcal vaccines. Vaccine impairment possible. Avoid most live vaccines.
- g.) Lung disease: For asthma, chronic obstruction pulmonary disease, active tuberculosis, cystic fibrosis, myasthenia gravis, chronic bronchitis and related conditions, recommend influenza and pneumococcal vaccines.
- h.) Spleen or bone marrow problems: If patient is asplenic or has bone marrow problems, recommend influenza, pneumococcal, Hib and meningococcal vaccines.
- i.) Weakened immune system: Recommend influenza and pneumococcal vaccines. Vaccine impairment is possible. Avoid most live vaccines. See detailed information about HIV infection; consider Hib vaccine.
- j.) Other: _________ Consider individually; refer to authoritative guidelines. If patient has chronic kidney disease (eg, dialysis,

transplant, erythropoetin therapy), cerebrospinal fluid leaks, chronic alcoholism, cirrhosis, sickle cell anemia, hepatic failure or some other chronic conditions, recommend influenza and pneumococcal vaccines. Hemophilia and thalassemia are indications for hepatitis B vaccine.

12.) What drugs or medications do you take? ____________________
Recommend influenza vaccine for children on chronic aspirin therapy. Other drugs often indicate an underlying chronic illness necessitating influenza, pneumococcal, hepatitis B or other vaccines (eg, insulin, theophylline, digoxin, coagulation factors).

13.) Are you exposed to blood, blood products or infectious materials? (circle one) No Yes
Recommend hepatitis B vaccine to those exposed to blood products (eg, healthcare workers, dialysis patients, hemophiliacs), as well as institutionalized mentally retarded, men who have sex with men, IV drug abusers, others.

Part II: To be completed by clinical personnel:

14.) Influenza A&B Vaccine History:
- a.) from oral history/from records (circle one)
- b.) date of most recent dose: ____________
- c.) vaccine last used: split-/whole-virion (circle one)
- d.) is today this patient's first dose?
  (circle one) No Yes Unknown
- e.) is a second dose needed? No Yes
  For people < 9 years old who have never received influenza vaccine before, give a second dose 1 month later. Use only split-virion vaccine for children ≤ 15 years old.

15.) Pneumococcal Vaccine History:
- a.) from oral history/from records (circle one)
- b.) previous dose? no data No Yes 14/23/?-valent
- c.) date of previous dose: ______________
  An additional dose of pneumococcal vaccine is recommended after 6 years for adults with asplenia, nephrotic syndrome or renal failure or transplant recipients. Revaccinate children with nephrotic syndrome, asplenia or sickle cell anemia after 3 to 5 years, if they would be ≤ 10 years old at revaccination.

16.) Tetanus-Diphtheria Toxoids History:
- a.) from oral history/from records (circle one)
- b.) basic series complete? No Yes No data
- c.) date of most recent dose: ____________
- d.) product last used: Plain tetanus toxoid (TT); adult-strength Td; pediatric-strength DT; DTwP; DTaP; unknown
  If basic series not complete, give needed doses. If most recent tetanus-diphtheria dose was > 10 years ago, give Td.

17.) Tuberculin Skin History:
- a.) date of most recent test: ____________
- b.) reaction: ____ mm × ____ mm/No reaction
- c.) old tuberculin (OT, Tine, MonoVacc)/ ___ tu PPD
  If the patient is tuberculin-negative, recommend a new test

for newly arrived immigrants, new residents of nursing homes, new prison inmates and employees of nursing homes and hospitals.

18.) Other Immunization Needs: Consider hepatitis A and B, measles, mumps, rubella, varicella, polio, Hib, rabies, others. Ask about international travel, occupation, lifestyle and other risk factors.

Part III: Immunization Order:

	Dose:	Route:	Site:	Lot #:	Admin By:	Date:
19.) Influenza Vaccine: Split/Whole	___ ml	IM	___	___	___	___
20.) Pneumococcal Vaccine:	___ ml	IM/SC	___	___	___	___
21.) Tetanus/Diphtheria: Adult Td, ped DT	___ ml	IM	___	___	___	___
22.) Tuberculin Test: OT/PPD	___ tu	ID	___	___	___	___
23.) Other: ___	___ ml	___	___	___	___	___
24.) Other: ___	___ ml	___	___	___	___	___

Use these blocks to record ordered doses by indicating product volume. For influenza, tetanus-diphtheria and tuberculin, a product choice must be made. Then record doses administered: Volume, site, lot number, name of person administering the dose and date.

25.) Ordered by: ___ Date: ___
Signature of prescriber authorizing these immunologic agents.

Part IV: Clinical Observations:

26.) Immediate reactions to these vaccines: ___
Date/Time noted: ___ Delayed: ___
Record immediate- and delayed-hypersensitivity reactions here. Note date and time of onset of reaction.

27.) Reaction to this tuberculin test: ___ mm × ___ mm
Read by: ___ Date read: ___

28.) Remarks: ___

This model form is provided as a service. This form may be freely reproduced for individual patients if credit is given to: Grabenstein JD. *Immunization Delivery: A Complete Guide.* St. Louis: Facts and Comparisons, 1997:(page).

Patient Identification Stamp Imprint

Immunizations may be recorded in the progress, treatment or encounter sections of a medical record, but data retrieval is more efficient if a dedicated form is used to record all immunizations, rather than having them interspersed among other medical records.

For example, federal hospitals and clinics use Standard Form (SF) 601, Immunization Record, as the common document for ambulatory charts. The American College of Physicians advocates a similar form they call the Patient Immunization Record Form.[8]

Even the position of immunization documents within a medical record is important. Moving a health-maintenance inventory, including recommendations for routine adult immunizations, to the front of an encounter record can increase vaccine delivery.[9]

While paper records are effective, electronic records offer advantages of speed, more complete retrieval and automated screening. Several studies have shown the value of automatic reminder messages, introspective medical records and screening by diagnosis or drug therapy for indicators of influenza or pneumococcal vaccine to increase vaccine delivery.[10-15]

Under the National Childhood Vaccine Injury Act (NCVIA) of 1986, all practices that immunize must record key immunization data for vaccines covered under the Act. The NCVIA is discussed in detail in chapter 9 on "Legal and Liability Issues." These include any vaccine containing antigens against diphtheria, tetanus, pertussis, measles, mumps, rubella, poliovirus or other vaccines added later (eg, *Haemophilus influenzae* type b, varicella, hepatitis B). To comply with the NCVIA, the data may be recorded in the patient's medical record or in an immunization log for the site of delivery. The data recorded, at a minimum, must include patient name, date of administration, vaccine manufacturer, antigen name, lot number and provider's name, address and title. It is good practice to keep a log of all vaccinations given.[1,16-17]

Clinics and hospitals have adopted a variety of mechanisms to satisfy this requirement. These include simple logs, rubber stamps or adhesive labels for pages of medical records and computer databases.[18-19]

Consider immunization logs to be permanent records. Do not purge them, whether they are written or electronic. Immunization records can be automated in simple databases (eg, *DBase, Foxpro, Microsoft Access*) or in more sophisticated databases integrated with other clinical functions (eg, prescription profiles, drug-interaction screening).

Several options are available for recording immunizations electronically. Dedicated programs have been written, such as *VacTrac* (SmithKline Beecham), *Vaccine Information Program* (VIP; Merck Vaccine Division) and Clinic Assessment Software Application (CASA). *VacTrac* and *VIP* are available from representatives of the vaccine manufacturers. CASA is distributed by the CDC's National Immunization Program. CASA can generate postcards encouraging immunization delivery. Revised versions of these software programs are released periodically.

Another option is to use various brands of prescription-profiling software commonly available in pharmacies. Never discard immunization records from a pharmacy's retrievable records. Depending on the software, assign recorded immunizations a unique series of "prescription" numbers to facilitate prolonged archiving. Electronic records also make it easier to screen immunization files for needed booster doses or to screen prescription files for drugs that suggest immunization indications. For example, prescriptions for digoxin, nitroglycerin, warfarin, theophylline, beta- adrenergic agonists, insulin, oral hypoglycemic agents and other drugs indicate heart disease, lung disease, diabetes and other diseases. These and other diagnoses are indications for annual influenza and periodic pneumococcal immunization.[14-15] See chapter 2 on "Too Many Deaths, Too Much Disease" for more details.

When querying people about their immunization history, memory cues can help them remember when they were vaccinated. For tetanus-diphtheria boosters, ask people about their last visit to an emergency room to treat a wound. To establish timing, ask whether vaccinations occurred before or after major life events (eg, births, marriages, deaths). If time is available for more thorough inquiry, ask the patient's family to check records that may be kept at home. Encourage people to bring family vaccine records to all medical visits.

Despite your best efforts in taking immunization histories, doubt will often persist. In many cases, people should be vaccinated in the face of doubt.[2,20-21] Risk of infection usually outweighs the risk of an adverse event in an immune person receiving vaccine. There is no danger in raising antibody levels higher when vaccinating an immune person.

An accompanying table on the following page summarizes data elements to include in the optimal immunization record. The broad categories of data encompass the patient's demographic characteristics, clinical data, travel history and immunization history.

If the immunization is given by someone other than the patient's primary healthcare provider, report the immunization to that primary-care provider by telephone or mail. This provides for continuity of care and avoids a patch-work of records. If the patient has no regular healthcare provider, refer the patient to one for additional care as needed, according to local practice standards. In either case, report all immunizations to any state or other immunization registries. For example, if state-supplied vaccines are used, inform the local health department on a regular basis. Follow the local procedures for your health department.

Despite all precautions to the contrary, adverse events temporally associated with immunization occur rarely. To monitor the safety of vaccines, the Food & Drug Administration (FDA) and CDC rely on health professionals to report adverse events. The Vaccine Adverse Events Reporting System (VAERS) took effect in November 1990, replacing separate systems at CDC (the obsolete Form 7119) and FDA (Form 1639). The MedWatch form is used to report adverse events for other immunologic drugs. These forms are discussed in chapter 6 on "Immunization Administration."

Optimal Data Elements for Immunization Profiles

Demographic Data:

- Patient name
- Gender
- Date of birth
- Occupation
- Telephone number
- Identification number
- Primary physician(s)

Clinical Data:

- Previous hypersensitivity reactions, allergies or serum sickness
- Pregnancy, current or planned
- Fever
- Any immunodeficiency in household
- Previous positive tuberculin skin test
- Medications taken regularly
- Any chronic illness

Travel History:

- International travel concluded
- International travel planned

Immunization History Table:

- Vaccine names along one axis
- Each vaccine dose along other axis
- Dose, site, route of administration
- Date given
- Manufacturer and lot number
- Date next dose due
- Reactions noted (local or systemic)

Clinic Immunization Record

Patient Immunization Record

Patient Name: ____________ Gender: ________________ Occupation: ______________

Identification #: ________________________________ Birth Date: ______________

Daytime Telephone #: ____

Previous Hypersentivity Reaction to:

Agent: _______________ Describe Reaction: ________ When? ______________

Agent: _______________ Describe Reaction: ________ When? ______________

Healthcare Provider(s): ____

Address: ____

Phone: ____

Ask each patient about: Pregnancy, fever, regular medications, chronic illness, previous reactions, travel plans, immunodeficiency in household.

Immunologic drug	Dose, site route of administration	Date given	Manufacturer	Lot #	Name, title of person giving drug	Date next dose due	Note
DTP,							5 doses
Dt, or							5 doses
Td							q10y
Haemophilus							
influenzae b							
Pneumococcal							all > 65y
Influenza							all > 65y
Measles							2 doses
Mumps							if > 1957
Rubella							
OPV							4 doses
eIPV							
Hepatitis B							3 doses
Tuberculin							Reaction:
Skin Test							
Other Vaccines:							

This model form is provided as a service. This form may be freely reproduced for individual patients, if credit is given to: Grabenstein JD. *Immunization Delivery: A Complete Guide.* St. Louis: Facts and Comparisons, 1997:101.

Informed-Consent Documents

Immunization usually involves giving an exogenous medication to a healthy person. While modern vaccines are effective and safe, rare adverse events of high consequence occur. For this reason, obtaining informed consent is recommended and, in some cases, required by law. The rationale and method for obtaining consent is discussed in chapter 4 on "Making Vaccine Decisions."[22-23]

Before injection, take precautions to prevent adverse events. This includes a review of the patient's history for possible hypersensitivity to the vaccine or its components. Inform the patient, his or her parent or guardian about any significant adverse reactions expected after vaccine administration. Obtain and record informed consent. Ask parents and guardians to inform the clinician of any events that occur.

For minors and incompetent adults, the categories of people who may legally provide informed consent are defined by state law and precedent. Often, this will include parents, stepparents, grandparents, adult brothers or sisters, adult aunts or uncles and other representatives with written authorization. Consult local authorities for guidance.

Standard information designed by the CDC is generally available from local health departments.

Vaccine Records For Patients

A patient's personal immunization record should span inpatient and outpatient immunization experiences. It also fills in the gaps if clinic records are lost. Several personal immunization records are available, including Public Health Service (PHS) Form 731, International Certificates of Vaccination, commonly called the "yellow shot record."[1] PHS Form 731 is used to document vaccines needed for international travel but it can also serve as a convenient document for a life's worth of vaccinations. PHS Form 731 is used by US military services for soldiers, sailors, airmen, marines, coast guardsmen and their family members (including reservists). It is also used by the US State Department for diplomats and their families. PHS Form 731 is available from the Government Printing Office (GPO, telephone 202-783-3238, stock number 017-001-00-440-5). Volume discounts are available. PHS Form 731 also may be available at local health departments.

Additionally, each state and the District of Columbia prints its own uniform immunization record card. These record cards are often designed for both pediatric and adult immunizations, again providing lifelong records.

Encourage people to take vaccine records to every healthcare visit. In Canada and several states, people are encouraged to keep their personal immunization records in their wallets.[24]

The electronics revolution may soon popularize "smart cards." Smart cards are portable electronic medical records the size of credit cards. As these miniature patient databases are developed and refined, dedicated immunization sections should be included in their design.

Lost Records

What if someone loses a vaccination record? Do you start all over with dose #1 of every needed vaccine? Ask the patient or parents to check with previous healthcare providers, daycare centers, schools and other sites that may have records.

CDC recommends not assuming that events occurred if no documents can confirm it. Vaccinate these people to be sure. Duplicated doses might result in a sore arm, but that is preferable to being susceptible to a potentially fatal disease.

Synthesis

To document immunizations, you may want to start by updating or reconstructing your own personal immunization record and those of your family. Local health departments can provide forms used in your area.

When you interview computer vendors, ask for software that allows electronic immunization tracking. Useful specifications include vaccine-drug interaction screening, efficient searching of files for diagnoses or prescription drugs and separate immunization data files that cannot be erased.

Infection-control committees and occupational-health departments can recommend or revise separate immunization records for the medical record. They can adopt screening forms for taking immunization histories and establish uniform policies for where, when, how, by whom and for whom immunization assessments occur. In other settings, medical forms or patient-need inventories can include specific items querying history of routine vaccinations (eg, influenza, pneumococcal, hepatitis B, tetanus-diphtheria, measles-mumps-rubella vaccines). Electronic systems can be designed to display reminder messages to increase immunization rates.

References

[1] Grabenstein JD. Get it in writing: Documenting immunizations. *Hosp Pharm* 1991;26:901-4.

[2] Temianka D, Fedson DS. Pneumococcal vaccination: When in doubt, go ahead. *JAMA* 1991;265:211-2.

[3] Preblud SR, Gross F, Halsey NA, et al. Assessment of susceptibility to measles and rubella. *JAMA* 1982;247:1134-7.

[4] Scott RMcN, Butler AB, Schydlower M, et al. Ineffectiveness of historical data in predicting measles susceptibility. *Pediatrics* 1984;73:777-80.

[5] Le CT. Parental knowledge of their own immunization to poliomyelitis. *JAMA* 1985;254:608-9 (letter).

[6] Murray DL, Lunch MA. Determination of immune status to measles, rubella, and varicella-zoster viruses among medical students: Assessment of historical information. *Am J Public Health* 1988;78:836-8.

[7] Grabenstein JD. *ImmunoFacts: Vaccines & Immunologic Drugs*. St. Louis: Facts and Comparisons, Inc., May 1997.

[8] American College of Physicians. *Guide for Adult Immunization,* 3rd ed. Philadelphia: American College of Physicians, 1994.

[9] Rodney WMacM, Chapivsky P, Quan M. Adult immunization: The medical record design as a facilitator for physician compliance. *J Med Educ* 1983;58:576-80.

[10] Brink SG. Provider reminders: Changing information format to increase infant immunizations. *Med Care* 1989;27:648-53.

[11] McDonald CJ, Hui SL, Smith DM, et al. Reminders to physicians from an introspective computer medical record. *Ann Intern Med* 1984;100:130-8.

[12] Klachko DM, Wright DL, Gardner DW. Effect of a microcomputer-based registry on adult immunizations. *J Fam Pract* 1989;29:169-72.

[13] Barton MB, Schoenbaum SC. Improving influenza vaccination performance in an HMO setting: The use of computer-generated reminders and peer comparison feedback. *Am J Publ Health* 1990;80:534-6.

[14] Grabenstein JD, Hayton B. Pharmacoepidemiologic program for identifying patients in need of vaccination. *Am J Hosp Pharm* 1990;47:1774-80.

[15] Grabenstein JD, Hartzema AG, Guess HA, et al. Community pharmacists as immunization advocates: A clinical pharmacoepidemiologic experiment. *Internat J Pharm Pract* 1993;2:5-10.

[16] Clayton EW, Hickson GB. Compensation under the National Childhood Vaccine Injury Act. *J Pediatr* 1990;116:508-13.

[17] Grabenstein JD. Compensation for vaccine injury: Balancing society's need and personal risk. *Hosp Pharm* 1995;30:831-2,834-6.

[18] Centers for Disease Control. National Childhood Vaccine Injury Act: Requirements for permanent vaccination records and for reporting of selected events after vaccination. *MMWR* 1988;37:197-200.

[19] Perkins LD. Complying with the National Childhood Vaccine Injury Act. *Am J Hosp Pharm* 1990;47:1260,1262,1266.

[20] Canadian Advisory Committee on Immunization. Statement on immunization of children with inadequate immunization records. *Can Dis Wkly Rpt* 1990;16(2):11-2.

[21] Snow R, Babish JD, McBean AM. Is there any connection between a second pneumonia shot and hospitalization among Medicare beneficiaries? *Publ Health Reports* 1995;110:720-5.

[22] Fulginiti VA. Patient education for immunizations. *Pediatrics* 1984;74(S):961-3.

[23] Landwirth J. Medical-legal aspects of immunization: Policy and practices. *Pediatr Clin N Amer* 1990;37:771-84.

[24] Canadian National Advisory Committee on Immunizations. *Canadian Immunization Guide,* 4th ed. Ottawa: Ministry of National Health & Welfare, 1993. Updated by fax: 613-941-3900.

CHAPTER 8

Administrative Issues

Facility Design

In most settings, little facility modification is needed to offer immunizations. Pharmacies that offer immunizations typically use counseling areas or waiting rooms to administer injections. In some cases, privacy is appropriate if people need to remove or adjust clothing to free the injection site. Redesign also may help muffle noises.

Practices just beginning to expand their immunization program may need to purchase screens or furniture to accommodate their new functions. Practices that adopt the educational role should assess the signs, posters and other messages seen by vaccinees.

Arrange the physical space to allow for fainting without injury. Position vaccinees near a hard surface in case cardiopulmonary resuscitation is needed.

Have the refrigerator and freezer near a flat counter top to allow for ease in dose preparation. Allow adequate storage space for consumable supplies and syringe disposal containers.

Marketing Issues

Most practices start slowly and allow signs and word of mouth to develop the clientele. Newspaper advertisements, flyers and posters for influenza programs are common.

When dealing with managed healthcare organizations, remember that immunization delivery is monitored in Health Plan Employer Data & Information Set (HEDIS) scores. It is a kind of report card employers use to compare managed care organizations. Offer to help managed care organizations improve their HEDIS score by increasing childhood, adolescent and adult immunization delivery.

Other Management Issues

After administering live, attenuated bacterial or viral products, treat all equipment and materials used as infectious waste. Incinerate, sterilize or dispose of them as biohazardous waste. Do not separate syringes from needles. Do not recap or clip needles. Use "sharps" containers; do not empty or reuse them. Replace them when they are ⅔ full. Hire a contractor to haul away "sharps" containers. Consider state regulations regarding biohazard disposal.

Occupational Safety & Health Administration (OSHA) regulations require universal precautions and body substance isolation for anyone potentially exposed to blood or other body fluids. Treat all body fluids as if infected. In this way, all blood-borne pathogens can be stopped.

OSHA requires that hepatitis B vaccine be offered without charge to any employee with potential contact to blood products (29 CFR 1910.1030(f)). If an at-risk employee chooses to decline hepatitis B vaccination, he or she is required by OSHA regulation to sign a specific informed declination: "I understand that due to my occupational exposure to blood or other potentially infectious materials I may be at risk of acquiring hepatitis B virus (HBV) infection. I have been given the opportunity to be vaccinated with hepatitis B vaccine at no charge to myself. However, I decline hepatitis B vaccination at this time. I understand that by declining this vaccine, I continue to be at risk of acquiring hepatitis B, a serious disease. If in the future I continue to have occupational exposure to blood or other potentially infectious materials, and I want to be vaccinated with hepatitis B vaccine, I can receive the vaccination series at no charge to me" (29 CFR 1910.1030 Appendix A). The regulations list other details to observe.

Obtaining Compensation

Compensation for administering immunizations comes from a variety of sources. In many settings, the value of vaccination is so obvious that people pay cash for the service. In some cases, you or they can seek reimbursement from their health insurance plan. Some vaccines are paid for by federal or state governments.

The federal Vaccines For Children (VFC) (42 USC 1396(S)) program pays for some pediatric vaccines. To be eligible to receive immunization through VFC, a child must be enrolled in Medicaid, have no health insurance, have health insurance without vaccine benefits or be an American Indian or Alaskan native. VFC covers any vaccine containing these antigens: diphtheria, tetanus, pertussis, measles, mumps, rubella, Hib, poliovirus or hepatitis B. Clinicians may charge a modest administration fee, but no child may be turned away for inability to pay that fee. VFC sites must agree to auditing of storage, handling, documentation and administrative procedures and to report utilization statistics.

Other state and federal funds may cover vaccines administered at local health departments or city or county health clinics. A few states pay for all vaccines for all children. Medicare Part B, the ambulatory portion of that program, reimburses its beneficiaries for three immunizations: Influenza, pneumococcal and hepatitis B vaccines (42 CFR 410.10, 410.57, 410.63 and 42 USC 1395). Immunization Practices Advisory Committee (ACIP) guidelines must be fulfilled. This reimbursement can even be made to hospitals for inpatients, despite the usual outpatient nature of Part B payments.

The steps for obtaining reimbursement from Medicare for immunization are described in the accompanying table on the following page. Medicare reimbursement rates vary from one location to another but are always based on two components: Vaccine price plus an administration fee. For example, in Mississippi in 1996, the administration fees were $3.07 in rural settings and $3.26 in urban settings. Allowable product costs were $3.37 for a dose of influenza vaccine, $11.90 for pneumococcal vaccine and $56.01 for hepatitis B vaccine. Rates may be higher or lower in other states.[1-2]

Medicare Reimbursement for Immunization

Here are key points in Medicare policies for billing for vaccination reimbursement. They are based on information provided by the Health Care Financing Administration (HCFA), the federal agency that implements the Medicare and Medicaid programs.[1-2] For detailed information, contact HCFA or your local Medicare carrier or intermediary.

1.) Obtain a Medicare provider or supplier number by contacting your local Medicare Part B carrier. Submit the required form, often HCFA Form 855, Provider/Supplier Enrollment Application. Allow 3 to 5 weeks for processing. Then obtain HCFA Form 1500 claim forms. These forms are available from the US Government Printing Office at 202-512-1800, which accepts credit cards for payment. The single-sheet version, stock number 01706000468-1, costs $9 per package of 100. Other formats are also available. Many third-party payers use HCFA Form 1500 as well.

2.) Coverage of influenza, pneumococcal and hepatitis B vaccines is available under Medicare Part B, regardless of the delivery setting. Medicare pays the entire cost of the vaccine and its administration.

3.) For its own administrative purposes, Medicare does not require that influenza vaccine be ordered by a physician. This policy does not negate other applicable state law or other requirements. Medicare does require a physician's order for pneumococcal or hepatitis B vaccine. However, a physician does not need to be present if a previously written order is on hand. Pneumococcal vaccination must involve:
   - Determining the person's age, health and vaccination status;
   - Obtaining a signed informed consent document;
   - Administering the vaccine only to people at high risk of pneumococcal disease who have not been previously vaccinated; and
   - Providing a record of vaccination to the vaccinee.

4.) Billing Forms:
   - Carrier Billing: Individual immunizations are billed on HCFA Form 1500. If the provider accepts Medicare payment as payment in full, there is no charge to the beneficiary. Electronic billing is feasible in some settings.
   - When five or more qualifying immunizations are administered on the same day by the same provider they may be billed on a single HCFA Form 1500 as "roster billing." Preprinted standardized information about the provider or supplier may be provided on the form, with rosters attached that contain the variable information needed for processing each claim. These rosters must include provider name, provider billing number, date of service, each vaccinee's Medicare health insurance claim number, last name, first name, middle name, date of birth and gender. Include the vaccinee's address if required by the contractor.

- Independent Rural Health Clinics (RHCs) and freestanding Federally Qualified Health Centers (FQHCs) bill according to Section 614 of the RHC/FQHC manual.
- Other providers bill for a vaccine and its administration on HCFA Form 1450, using revenue code 636 for the vaccine and 771 for the administration fee, plus the diagnosis and HCPCS codes. HCPCS, pronounced hik-piks, is an acronym for HCFA's Common Procedure Coding System. Roster billing with HCFA Form 1450 is also permitted.
- Provider facilities not participating in Medicare (eg, nursing homes) are considered suppliers and bill their local carrier. The Part B carrier issues supplier numbers upon request.
- Entities such as chain drug stores that meet state requirements to administer vaccine may bill local carriers as suppliers.
- Self-employed nurses licensed under state law to immunize may obtain provider numbers and bill local carriers.
- Beneficiaries enrolled in Medicare-contracted health maintenance organizations (HMOs) may be required to obtain immunization through their plan provider. Otherwise, they may have to pay for it out-of-pocket. HMO enrollees can check with their plan to see if they are "locked-in" in this way. If not locked in, they may be immunized by any qualified provider.
- HMOs that immunize non-member Medicare beneficiaries are treated as suppliers and bill the carrier. Specialty code 99 is acceptable for an HMO.

5.) Billing Codes:

	ICD-9-CM Diagnosis Code[1]	CPT Procedure Code[2]	HCPCS Code for Medicare HCFA Billing[3]
Influenza vaccine	V04.8	90724	G0008
Pneumococcal vaccine	V03.82	90732	G0009
Hepatitis B vaccine (adult) [alternate listing]	V05.3	90746 90731	G0010
BCG vaccine	V03.2	90728	
Cholera vaccine	V03.0	90725	
Diphtheria-tetanus toxoids pediatric (DT)	V06.8	90702	
Diphtheria-tetanus-acellular pertussis vaccine (DTaP)	V06.8	90700	
Diphtheria-tetanus-whole cell pertussis vaccine (DTwP)	V06.1	90701	
DTwP-*Haemophilus influenzae* type B (Hib) vaccines	V06.8	90720	
DTwP-poliovirus vaccine	V06.3	90711	
Haemophilus influenzae type b (Hib) vaccine	V03.81	90737	
Hepatitis A vaccine	V05.3	90730	
Hepatitis B vaccine (11-19 y/o)	V05.3	90745	G0010
Hepatitis B vaccine (birth to 10 y/o)	V05.3	90744	G0010

	ICD-9-CM Diagnosis Code[1]	CPT Procedure Code[2]	HCPCS Code for Medicare HCFA Billing[3]
Hepatitis B vaccine (dialysis or immunosuppressed patient)	V05.3	90747	G0010
Measles vaccine	V04.2	90705	
Measles-mumps-rubella vaccine	V06.4	90707	
Measles-mumps-rubella-varicella vaccine	V06.8	90710	
Measles-rubella vaccine	V06.8	90708	
Meningococcal vaccine, any formulation	V03.89	90733	
Mumps vaccine	V04.6	90704	
Mumps-rubella vaccine	V06.8	90709	
Plague vaccine	V03.3	90727	
Poliovirus vaccine, injectable	V04.0	90713	
Poliovirus vaccine, oral	V05.8	90712	
Rabies vaccine	V04.5	90726	
Rubella vaccine	V04.3	90706	
Tetanus toxoid	V03.7	90703	
Tetanus-diphtheria toxoids adult (Td)	V06.8		
Typhoid vaccine	V03.1	90714	
Varicella vaccine	V05.4	90716	
Yellow-fever vaccine	V04.4	90717	
Immune globulin intramuscular (see ICD-9-CM Code book)	V03.0-V06.9	90741	
Hyperimmune globulins (eg, hepatitis B, rabies, $Rh_o(D)$, tetanus, vaccinia, varicella-zoster (see ICD-9-CM Code book)	V03.0-V06.9	90742	
Specified vaccine NEC (see ICD-9-CM Code book)	V03.0-V06.9		
Vaccination not carried out because of contraindication	V64.0		

[1] The reason for the visit according to the International Classification of Diseases, 9th edition, Clinical Modification.

[2] The Current Procedural Terminology (CPT) code for administering the vaccine. Not used for billing Medicare.

[3] The HCPCS Level II code ("national code") for administering the vaccine, used for billing Medicare only. Medicare presently reimburses for three vaccines only.

Questions and Answers About Medicare's Influenza Vaccination Benefits[3]

Coverage Policy

Q. What individuals and entities may bill Medicare for the influenza vaccine and its administration?
A. For the influenza vaccination benefit, any individual or entity meeting state licensure requirements may qualify to have payment made for furnishing and administering influenza vaccine to Medicare beneficiaries enrolled under Part B.

Q. Does a physician have to be present during immunization? Is a physician order (written or verbal), plan of care or any other type of physician involvement required for Medicare coverage of flu shots?
A. Medicare does not require a physician to be present. However, the law in individual states may require a physician. Physician involvement is not required for Medicare coverage; however, individual state law may require a physician order or other physician involvement.

Q. There has been some confusion about how often a beneficiary can receive a flu shot and have it covered by Medicare. If a beneficiary receives a flu shot more than once in a 12-month period, will Medicare still pay for it?
A. Generally, Medicare pays for one flu shot per flu season. This may mean that a beneficiary will receive more than one flu shot in a 12-month period. For example, a beneficiary may receive a flu shot in January 1996 for the 1995-96 flu season and another flu shot in October 1996 for the 1996-97 flu season. In this case, Medicare will pay for both flu shots because the beneficiary received only one flu shot per flu season.

Q. What if a beneficiary needs more than one flu shot in a flu season?
A. Medicare will pay for more than one flu shot per flu season if it is reasonable and medically necessary.

Q. Is a person with only Part A coverage entitled to receive the flu shot and have it covered under Part B?
A. No. The influenza vaccine and its administration are a Part B-covered service only.

Q. What types of nontraditional providers and suppliers may bill a carrier for flu shots?
A. If they meet state licensure requirements to furnish and administer influenza vaccinations, individuals and entities that may obtain a Medicare provider number and bill Medicare include but are not limited to: Drug stores, senior centers, shopping malls and self-employed nurses. These providers and suppliers should contact their local contractor to receive a provider number.

Q. May a registered nurse employed by a physician use the physician's provider number if the nurse provides flu shots in a location other than the physician's office?
A. If the nurse is not working for the physician when the services are provided (eg, a nurse is administering flu shots at a shopping mall at his or her own direction and not that of the physician), the nurse may obtain a

provider number and bill the carrier directly. However, if the nurse is working for the physician when the services are provided, the nurse would use the physician's provider number.

Q. What types of providers may bill the intermediary for the influenza and pneumococcal pneumonia vaccines?
A. The following providers may bill intermediaries for this benefit:

- Hospitals;
- Skilled Nursing Facilities (SNFs);
- Christian Science Sanatoriums (CSSs);
- Rural Primary Care Hospitals (RPCHs);
- Home Health Agencies (HHAs);
- Comprehensive Outpatient Rehabilitation Facilities (CORFs);
- Rural Health Clinics (RHCs);
- Federally Qualified Health Centers (FQHCs);
- Outpatient Physical Therapy (OPT) providers; and
- Independent Renal Dialysis Facilities (RDFs).

Q. Will Medicare pay an HHA for a nurse's visit when he or she goes into a patient's home to furnish the flu vaccine?
A. Where the sole purpose for an HHA visit is to administer a vaccine (influenza, PPV, or hepatitis B), Medicare will not pay for a skilled nursing visit by an HHA nurse under the HHA benefit. However, the vaccine and its administration is covered under the vaccine benefit. The administration should include charges only for the supplies being used and the cost of the injection. HHA's are not permitted to charge for travel time or other expenses (eg, gasoline).

Payment Policy

Q. Is a coinsurance payment or deductible required for the flu vaccine benefit?
A. No. Medicare pays 100% of the Medicare approved charge or the submitted charge, whichever is lower. Neither the $100 annual deductible nor the 20% coinsurance apply. Therefore, if a beneficiary receives a flu shot from a physician, provider or supplier that agrees to accept assignment (eg, agrees to accept Medicare payment as payment in full), there is no cost to the beneficiary. If a beneficiary receives a flu shot from a physician, provider or supplier that does not accept assignment, the physician may collect his or her usual charge.

Q. May providers, physicians and suppliers charge and collect payment from Medicare beneficiaries for the flu shot?
A. Nonparticipating physicians, providers and suppliers that do not accept assignment may collect payment from the beneficiary, but they must submit an unassigned claim on the beneficiary's behalf. Participating institutional physicians, providers and suppliers that accept assignment must bill Medicare if they charge a fee to cover any or all costs related to the provision or administration of the influenza vaccine. They may not collect payment from beneficiaries.

Q. Does the limiting charge provision apply to the flu benefit?
A. No. Nonparticipating physicians and suppliers that do not accept assign-

ment for the flu benefit may collect their usual charges (eg, the amount charged a patient who is not a Medicare beneficiary) for influenza vaccine and its administration. The beneficiary is responsible for paying the difference between what the physician or supplier charges and the amount Medicare allows.

Q. Why doesn't limiting charge apply to influenza vaccine administration?
A. Only items and services paid through the Physician Fee Schedule (and certain other items and services as specified by Congress) are subject to the statutory limiting charge limits. Influenza vaccine and its administration are neither paid through the Physician Fee Schedule nor otherwise covered under the limiting charge provision of the law. A change in Medicare law would be required for influenza vaccine and its administration to be covered under the limiting charge provision.

Q. Does the 5% payment reduction for physicians who do not accept assignment apply to the flu shot benefit?
A. No. Only items and services covered under limiting charge are subject to the 5% payment reduction.

Q. Why is there such a variation between states and within states in Medicare reimbursement rates for flu vaccine and its administration?
A. Medicare's allowed payment amount for influenza vaccine is determined as it is for any other drug (eg, Medicare pays the lower of the actual charge or the median average wholesale price [AWP]). Therefore, a provider whose actual charge is the same as the AWP will receive the AWP, and a provider whose actual charge is less than the AWP will receive the lower payment. The payment rate for flu vaccine for each carrier is simply the average of all payments for the vaccine made in that carrier's locality. Therefore, each carrier's payment rate varies depending upon how many providers have charged less than the AWP. Medicare payment by carriers for the administration of the vaccine is linked to payment for services under the physician fee schedule but is not actually paid under the physician fee schedule. The charge for the administration is the lesser of the actual charge or the fee schedule amount for a comparable injection. Because fee schedules are adjusted for each Medicare payment locality, there is a variation in the payment amount nationwide. Intermediary payment to a provider for the influenza vaccine and its administration is made on the basis of reasonable cost.

Q. Why can't Medicare pay one nationwide rate for flu shots?
A. The way in which Medicare pays for a given item or service is determined by statute. It would require congressional legislation for Medicare to pay a nationwide rate.

Q. May a physician, provider or supplier charge a Medicare beneficiary more for an immunization than he or she charges a non-Medicare patient?
A. No.

Q. If a beneficiary receives both flu and pneumococcal vaccines on the same day, will Medicare pay twice for the administration fee?
A. Yes.

Q. May a physician, provider or supplier collect payment for an immunization from a beneficiary and instruct the beneficiary to submit the claim to Medicare for payment?
A. No. Medicare law (Section 1848(g)(4) of the Social Security Act) requires that physicians, providers and suppliers submit a claim for services to Medicare on the beneficiary's behalf.

Q. Is HCPCS code G0008 (administration of influenza vaccine) subject to rebundling guidelines?
A. No. HCPCS code G0008 may be paid in addition to other services, including evaluation and management services.

Q. If a physician sees a beneficiary for the sole purpose of administering influenza vaccine, may he or she routinely bill for an office visit?
A. No. However if a patient actually receives other services constituting an "office visit" level of service, the physician may bill for a visit and Medicare will pay for the visit if it is reasonable and medically necessary.

Billing Medicare

Q. What information is needed on the HCFA-1450 and HCFA-1500 to bill for the influenza virus vaccine?
A. All data fields that are required for any Part B claim are required for the vaccine and its administration. Providers should bill according to the bill completion instructions in the various provider manuals.

Q. Who bills for the influenza vaccine when it is furnished to a dialysis patient of a hospital or hospital-based renal dialysis facility?
A. Regardless of where the vaccine is administered to a dialysis patient of a hospital, the hospital bills the intermediary using bill type 13X.

Q. What bill types are applicable for this benefit?
A. Applicable bill types are: 12X, 13X, 22X, 23X, 34X, 42X, 52X, 72X (independent RDFs only), 74X (OPTs only) and 75X.

Q. Independent RHCs must use revenue code 521 to bill. How should they show the charge for vaccine and administration on the HCFA-1450?
A. RHCs follow guidelines in Section 614 of the RHC/FQHC Manual. They do not include charges for the vaccine or its administration or the HCFA-1450. Payment is made at cost settlement.

Q. Are providers allowed to use therapy revenue codes on the flu vaccine claim?
A. Providers bill for the vaccine using revenue code 636 and for the administration using revenue code 771. If therapy services are also provided, they can be reflected on the same claim with the vaccine and its administration.

Q. Should Part A shared systems maintainers allow condition code "A6" or special program indicator "06" on vaccine claims?
A. Condition code A6 is used to indicate services not subject to deductible and coinsurance.

Q. For inpatient hospital and inpatient skilled nursing facilities, what revenue code is used for the administration?

A. All providers that bill the intermediary for the vaccine report the administration under revenue code 771.

Q. What bill type do hospitals and skilled nursing facilities report for inpatients who receive this benefit?
A. Hospitals bill for the vaccine under bill type 13X and report the date of discharge instead of the actual date of service unless they are using a roster bill. Hospitals using a roster bill may use the actual date of service. Skilled nursing facilities bill under bill type 22X.

Q. May other charges be listed on the same bill with the flu vaccine?
A. Yes. However, there must be separate coding for the additional charge(s).

Q. What should be entered in item 11 of the HCFA-1500 when Medicare is known to be the secondary payer?
A. For all influenza vaccination claims submitted to a carrier, item 11 of the preprinted HCFA-1500 should show "NONE."

Q. May certified Part A providers submit claims to a carrier?
A. No. Except for hospice providers, Part A providers must bill their intermediary for this Part B benefit. Hospice providers bill the carrier.

Q. How should nonparticipating facilities (eg, nursing homes) bill Medicare?
A. Non-Medicare-participating facilities bill their local carrier.

Q. May HHAs that have a Medicare-certified component and a non-Medicare-certified component elect to furnish the influenza benefit through the noncertified component and bill the Part B carrier?
A. Yes.

Claims Processing

Q. What if a provider or beneficiary submits a claim with the incorrect HCPCS code?
A. If the diagnosis code is V04.8 and the narrative description (if annotated on the claim) says "flu shot" but the HCPCS code is incorrect, change the HCPCS code and pay for the flu shot. However, if the incorrect code is not obviously wrong (eg, there is no narrative and the procedure and diagnosis codes do not agree), the carrier must follow the Medicare Carriers Manual, Part 3, Section 4020.

Q. How do carriers handle flu shot claims for Railroad Retirement Board (RRB) beneficiaries whose claims are normally forwarded to Metrahealth for processing?
A. Replicate the roster and the HCFA-1500, highlighting the RRB beneficiary on the roster, and forward the material to the appropriate Metrahealth-RRB processing center. (See Medicare Carriers Manual, Part 3, Sections 3103 and 3110.B.)

Q. How should carriers handle beneficiary-submitted flu claims?
A. Carriers should process these claims under procedures that are applied in other situations in which unassigned claims (HCFA-1490's) are received from beneficiaries. (See Medicare Carriers Manual, Part 3, Section 3042.) Carriers should use the provider-specific information included on receipts

submitted by beneficiaries to construct a skeleton provider record and assign a temporary provider number for the entity that furnished the service. Carriers should need minimal information to assign a provider number and establish/create a provider file record. Carriers should also initiate appropriate educational contacts with these entities concerning Medicare billing requirements for covered Part B services, obtain a formal provider application and assign a provider identification number.

Q. There has been some concern about the confusion caused by providers advertising flu shots as "free." When people later receive Explanation of Medicare Benefits (EOMBs), they contact the carrier to report fraudulent billing. Should providers advertise this as a free service?
A. Physicians, providers and suppliers that accept assignment may advertise that there will be no charge to the beneficiary, but they should make it clear that a claim will be submitted to Medicare on their behalf. Physicians, providers and suppliers that do not accept assignment should never advertise the service as free because there will be an out-of-pocket expense for the beneficiary after Medicare has paid 100% of the Medicare-allowed amount.

Edits

Q. Are there influenza edits in the Common Working File (CWF)?
A. Influenza edits will be installed in CWF soon. Some contractors have edits in their systems so claims for more than one flu shot in a flu season can be screened for medical necessity.

Q. Are claims for influenza vaccine and administration subject to Common Working File (CWF) Medicare Secondary Payer (MSP) edits?
A. CWF waives MSP development on carrier-processed flu claims when the only service on the claim is for the influenza virus vaccine and its administration. CWF also waives MSP development on roster-billed intermediary-processed claims. However, if a provider knows that a particular group health plan covers the influenza virus vaccine and its administration and all other MSP requirements for the Medicare beneficiary are met, the primary payer must be billed.

Mass Immunizers

Note: Although these questions primarily concern mass immunizers, they may apply to any entity immunizing Medicare beneficiaries.

Q. What is a mass immunizer?
A. As used by HCFA, a mass immunizer offers flu shots to many individuals (the public or members of a specific group, such as residents of a retirement community). Mass immunizers must accept assignment. Often the flu shots are offered during a special "flu program" or "flu clinic." A mass immunizer may be a traditional Medicare provider or supplier (such as a hospital outpatient department) or may be a nontraditional provider or supplier (such as a senior citizens' center or a public health clinic).

Q. May providers, physicians and suppliers submit claims for the flu benefit to Medicare if they provide the benefit free of charge or on a sliding fee scale to other patients?

A. Nongovernmental entities (providers, physicians or suppliers) that provide immunizations free of charge to all patients, regardless of their ability to pay, may not bill Medicare. (See Medicare Carriers Manual, Part 8, Section 2306.) However, a nongovernmental entity that does not charge patients who are unable to pay or reduces its charge for patients of limited means (sliding fee scale) but does expect to be paid if a patient has health insurance that covers the items or services provided, may bill Medicare and receive Medicare payment. State and local government entities (such as public health clinics) may bill Medicare for immunizations given to beneficiaries even if they provide immunizations free to all patients, regardless of their ability to pay.

Q. Historically, some entities that have provided mass immunization programs have not charged patients the full cost of the flu vaccine and its administration, because they have subsidized part of the cost from their budgets. Instead, they have requested a specific dollar "donation" that covers part of the cost of the flu shot. These entities do not submit a claim to Medicare for the beneficiary. Is this an acceptable practice?
A. No. Because the flu benefit does not require any beneficiary coinsurance or deductible, a Medicare beneficiary has a right to receive this benefit without incurring any out-of-pocket expense. Also, the entity is required by law to submit a claim to Medicare on behalf of the beneficiary.

The entity may bill Medicare for the amount that is not subsidized from its budget. For example, an entity that incurs a cost of $7.50 per flu shot and pays $2.50 of the cost from its budget may bill the carrier the $5.00 cost that is not paid out of its budget.

Q. Sometimes an entity receives donated flu vaccine or receives donated services for the administration of the vaccine. In these cases, may the provider bill Medicare for the portion of the flu shot that was not donated?
A. Yes.

Mass Immunizer Enrollment Process

Note: This enrollment process applies only to entities that will (1) bill a carrier; (2) use roster bills; and (3) bill only for flu shots.

Q. Do providers and suppliers that want to mass immunize and submit claims to Medicare on roster bills have to enroll in the Medicare program?
A. Yes. Providers and suppliers must enroll in Medicare even if mass immunizations are the only service they will provide to Medicare beneficiaries. They can enroll by filling out the HCFA-855, the Provider/Supplier Enrollment application. Providers and suppliers who wish to roster bill for mass immunizations should contact the Medicare contractor servicing their area for a copy of the enrollment application and special instructions for mass immunizers that will roster bill. Providers and suppliers who will not provide other covered services to Medicare beneficiaries complete only the portion of the form that applies to mass immunizers.

Q. If providers/suppliers enroll in Medicare to roster bill for mass immunizations only, may they bill Medicare for other Part B services?
A. No. Providers/Suppliers who wish to bill for other Part B services must enroll as a provider or supplier by completing the entire HCFA-855.

Q. Why enroll providers if they are going to provide mass immunizations to Medicare beneficiaries only once a year?
A. Although HCFA wants to make it as easy as possible for providers and suppliers to immunize Medicare beneficiaries and bill Medicare, it must ensure that those providers who wish to enroll in Medicare are qualified providers, receive a provider number and receive the proper payment.

Simplified Billing Procedures (Roster Billing)

Q. Is electronic billing available for roster-billed claims?
A. Yes. Contractors should have available low- or no-cost software for providers to use when roster billing electronically.

Q. How many beneficiaries per day must be vaccinated for the roster billing procedure to be used?
A. Generally, five beneficiaries per day must be vaccinated to roster bill. However, this requirement is waived for inpatient hospitals that mass immunize and use the roster billing method. This requirement also is waived for physicians who provide flu shots to patients in their offices.

Q. What specialty code should be used for public health clinics (PHCs) that bill carriers for influenza vaccine and its administration?
A. PHCs should use specialty code "60," public health or welfare agencies (federal, state and local).

Q. What specialty code should be used for entities other than PHCs when influenza vaccinations are the only Part B-covered service they provide?
A. Such entities should use the HCFA specialty code that best defines their provider type. If there is no appropriate HCFA specialty code for their provider type, these entities may use specialty code 99.

Q. What blocks on the HCFA-1500 can be preprinted for providers using roster billing for influenza virus vaccine and administration claims?
A. The following blocks can be preprinted on a HCFA-1500: Block 1 (Medicare); Block 2 (See Attached Roster); Block 11 (None); Block 20 (No); Block 21 (V04.8); Block 24B (71); Block 24D (90724 and G0008 [separate line items for each]); Block 26 (Yes); and Block 29 (0).

Q. Do providers show the charge for one service or the total for all patients in block 24F of the modified HCFA-1500?
A. Providers should show the unit cost because contractors will have to replicate the claim for each beneficiary listed on the roster.

Q. If a beneficiary receives a flu shot at a mobile unit, what place of service code should be used?
A. A PHC-affiliated mobile unit should use POS code "71." A mobile unit not affiliated with a PHC should use "99" (other).

Q. What information needs to be submitted on a patient roster form that will be attached to a preprinted HCFA-1500 under the simplified roster billing procedure?
A. The following should be included on the roster form: Patient Name; Health Insurance Claim Number; Date of Birth; Sex; Date of Service; Signature or stamped "Signature on File" (see following question); and Provider Identification Number.

The format of the beneficiary roster can be modified to meet the needs of individual providers. It is the responsibility of the carrier to develop suitable roster formats that meet provider and carrier needs and contain the minimum data necessary to satisfy claims processing requirements for these claims.

Q. Are there any circumstances under which a signature is not required on a roster bill submitted to a carrier? For example, what if an entity is unable to obtain a beneficiary's signature because of incompetence?
A. A signature on file stamp or notation qualifies as a signature on a roster claim form when the provider has access to a signature on file in the beneficiary's record (eg, when administered in a physician's office).

Q. What should the carrier do if a roster bill is received without a beneficiary's signature?
A. The carrier should not deny or reject influenza virus vaccination claims if there is no beneficiary signature submitted.

Q. May hospitals and other entities that bill intermediaries use the "signature on file" designation on a roster bill?
A. Yes. Inpatient/outpatient departments of hospitals and outpatient departments of other providers may use a signature on file stamp or notation if they have access to a signature on file in the beneficiaries record.

Q. If the Health Insurance Claim Number (HICN) is incorrect, will the contractor contact the provider or beneficiary to correct it?
A. The "Date of Birth" column on the roster should, with other data elements, provide sufficient beneficiary information to resolve incorrect HICNs. It is unlikely that providers will have any additional information that would be helpful. If additional information is needed, the contractor should contact the beneficiary.

Q. May other services be listed with the influenza vaccine and administration on the modified HCFA-1500?
A. No. Other covered services are subject to more comprehensive data requirements which the roster billing process is not designed to accommodate. Other services should be billed using normal Part B claims filing procedures and forms.

Q. In some instances, two entities, such as a grocery store and a pharmacy, jointly sponsor a flu shot clinic, and each is reluctant to accept responsibility for billing. What are the criteria for determining the responsible party?
A. Assuming that a charge is made for the vaccine and its administration, the entity that furnishes the vaccine and the entity that administers the vaccine are each required to submit claims. Both parties must file sepa-

rately for the component furnished for which a charge was made.

When billing only for the administration, billers should indicate in block 24 of the HCFA-1500 that they did not furnish the vaccine. For roster-billed claims, cross through the preprinted item 24 line item component that was not furnished by the billing entity or individual.

Q. Will the roster billing criteria be changed to include mass immunizers that do not accept assignment?
A. No. The decision to permit mass immunizers to roster bill was made to ensure that the beneficiaries would receive flu shots but would not incur out-of-pocket expenses.

Managed Care

Q. Health Maintenance Organizations (HMOs), under a risk contract with HCFA, provided the vaccine during a health fair to their members and other Medicare beneficiaries not enrolled in the HMO for a fee. How will these HMOs bill Medicare for flu vaccines administered to fee-for-service beneficiaries not enrolled in their HMO? Do carriers issue a provider number under the streamlined procedure and process the claims using the simplified process, coding the specialty designation as "99" (Unknown Physician Specialty)?
A. HMOs that furnish influenza vaccinations to nonmember Medicare beneficiaries bill the carrier. The carrier will issue a provider number to the HMO. Specialty code 99 is acceptable for an HMO. The HMO may use roster billing only if vaccinations are the sole Medicare-covered services furnished by the HMO to nonmember Medicare patients.

Q. Beneficiaries have difficulty distinguishing between cost and risk HMOs. What is the distinction between cost and risk HMOs? How does this affect the beneficiary?
A. Beneficiaries enrolled in a risk HMO, called "locked-in," must receive all of their care through the plan's doctors, hospitals and other healthcare providers, except emergency care and unforeseen out-of-area care.

Beneficiaries enrolled in a cost HMO may choose to receive all of their care through the plan's doctors, hospitals and other healthcare providers or from healthcare providers who participate in the Medicare program. However, if beneficiaries do not choose a plan healthcare provider, they are responsible for paying the coinsurance and deductibles associated with such care.

Q. What should carriers do if providers submit claims for beneficiaries who are "locked-in" to their HMO when the vaccine is furnished by a facility or provider outside their HMO?
A. Medicare will not reimburse a non-HMO provider for flu shots for beneficiaries enrolled in risk HMOs. Medicare has already paid the HMO to provide this service.

Q. If a beneficiary who belongs to a risk HMO receives a flu shot from a fee-for-service provider, who is responsible for the payment?
A. Beneficiaries will have to pay out-of-pocket for the shot.

Q. What should carriers do if these claims show up in their Quality Assurance (QA) sample?
A. Carriers should review QA sample influenza virus vaccine claims billed using the simplified billing process against the instructions provided in the implementing instructions.

Q. Is the beneficiary responsible for a co-payment when a vaccine is provided at HMOs where a co-payment is required for any office visit?
A. Yes. The HMO is permitted to charge a co-payment. However, HCFA has asked managed care plans to waive co-payments for flu shots.

Note: Contact HCFA or your local Medicare carrier for the most up-to-date information.

References

[1] Anonymous. How to get Medicare reimbursement for vaccinations. *Pharmacy Reimbursement & Disease Management Report* 1996;1(May):4-7.
[2] Lorenz EW, ed. *Coding & Reimbursement Guide for Pharmacists.* Reston, VA: St. Anthony Publishing, Inc., November 1996.
[3] Health Care Financing Administration, July 1, 1996.

CHAPTER 9

Legal and Liability Issues

Legal Issues

Under federal law, the Food Drug & Cosmetic Act prohibits dispensing any human vaccine, immune globulin or other immunologic drug without a prescription from a licensed prescriber.[1-2] In common practice, immunization programs have been sponsored by organizations or institutions with the concurrence of a physician where traditional individual physician-patient relationships do not exist.

Individual state laws govern healthcare practice. Each state adopts specific regulations regarding who may prescribe within the scope-of-practice for each health profession. Each state also determines who is granted authority to administer drugs.

Under provisions of the Food Drug & Cosmetic Act, manufacturers may only print in a drug's package insert uses of a drug for which adequate information scientifically establishes safety and efficacy. FDA approval establishes that adequate scientific evidence of safety and efficacy has been compiled. The FDA does not literally approve the use of drugs or regulate the practice of medicine or how prescribers use licensed drugs. The FDA does have the authority to limit promotion of a given drug to information listed in the FDA-approved product labeling.[3-6]

Professional Liability

Note: This section provides an overview of some laws and regulations associated with immunization. Legal issues are complex and vary from state to state. This brief review cannot cover every topic of the law. Do not consider this section to be legal advice. Address specific questions to your attorney before making personal or policy decisions.

The malpractice risks for healthcare providers who immunize are low. The risks are especially low for those who immunize children. In traditional and non-traditional settings, vaccine providers are protected by a strong set of legal provisions, but no law provides absolute protection to the individual.[2,6-9] The single best defense against liability is good training coupled with professional, competent performance. The cause of successful medical malpractice suits is almost always negligence by the provider. The primary questions for an attorney deciding whether to sue must be "Can I prove negligence?" and, if so, "Can I prove damages to my client?"

The private and public healthcare systems have immunized children for decades. Much of the current concern about increased liability is directed toward groups of people who have not been immunized in the past or to non-traditional locations for immunizations.

Immunizing ranks low among medical procedures by risk of causing litigation against a healthcare professional. Additionally, the professional is protected from personal liability by an extensive set of statutes in most states. Providers in a non-traditional setting will often be covered by one or more of the types of statutes described below.

The most important of these laws, which covers many vaccine-related injuries, is the National Vaccine Injury Compensation Program (VICP). VICP is a form of no-fault insurance against events listed in the Vaccine Injury Table (VIT). In exchange for simplified proceedings, petitioners give up the right to file claims for punitive damages or derivative (family) claims. If one of the events in the section below can be proven, the claimant will be awarded damages from a federal fund.

The VICP has the advantage of being national in scope. It is limited to children and adults immunized with vaccines containing antigens against diphtheria, tetanus, pertussis, measles, mumps, rubella and poliovirus. Hepatitis B, *Haemophilus influenzae* type b and varicella vaccines will probably be added to this list in 1997. Details about VICP are provided at the end of this chapter.

Protections Under State Law

Other vaccine liability protections arise in state law. These protections may take the form of immunity from civil liability or indemnification from damages awarded. Examples include these:

- People acting on the orders of the state health department.
- People acting as a service volunteer of a charitable organization.
- People administering or authorizing a vaccine required by law.
- People acting within the scope of duties of employment or volunteer services rendered on school premises.
- Title 42 of the US Code, Section 233 (42 USC 233), allows people acting with funding under one of four federal community health services programs to be indemnified by the Federal Tort Claims Act.

Workers' Compensation laws may come into play for an infection judged to be an occupational disease contracted on the job. Workers' Compensation provisions may limit awards for adverse reactions caused by a vaccine.

In some cases, willful or wrongful acts or acts of gross negligence will not be covered by these protections. In other cases, governmental units may be responsible for the negligent acts of their employees. Negligence might be alleged if the injection is given with a dirty or used needle, an inappropriate site is used, the wrong vaccine is given, the given vaccine is contraindicated or the provider failed to assess the vaccinee adequately.

Negligence is the breach of a duty of care. Healthcare professionals have a duty of care to administer vaccines with appropriate care and vigilance. Gross negligence is to act with conscious indifference to the rights of others. The CDC and other experts have explicitly stated a full physical examination is unwarranted before immunization. The questions outlined in the annotated screening form in chapter 7 on "Immunization Documentation" can help avoid claims of negligence of this type.

What happens if a government employee does volunteer immunization work with a private-sector agency? These and several other unusual circumstances are often not directly covered by state law. Only a court can definitively apply the law to the situation, but, given the importance of the public policy involved, courts have clear incentives to act to protect the public's health through immunization.

Healthcare providers cannot be sued while vaccine-injured children and their families pursue redress under VICP. Even so, providers can later be found negligent, such as in vaccinating without asking about contraindications.

Even if negligence does occur in a child's case, a plaintiff's attorney must first go through the procedure provided by VICP, where negligence will not be an issue. Most injured claimants will obtain satisfaction by this route, but if the attorney does file suit in state court, the attorney for the defendant can present a series of arguments in defense. One can argue that the injury was caused by the vaccine, that the defendant was not subject to liability, that a government entity should indemnify him or by other grounds provided by state law. A plaintiff rejecting the award of the VICP proceeding would have to pursue expensive and difficult litigation in state court, where the award of damages might prove elusive.

Business Liability

In general, private businesses do not subject themselves to increased liability by allowing their premises to be used for immunizations. The National Childhood Vaccine Injury Act offers some protection in this regard. This act protects those sued because of harm caused by the immunization. Under many state negligence laws, property owners are responsible for three classes of people: Trespassers, licensees and invitees. Children and their guardians seeking immunizations at malls or grocery stores would be classified as invitees, specifically business visitors. The normal duty of property owners is the same with immunizations as with everyday business–to inspect the premises for defects or dangerous conditions, then correct those dangers or warn invitees about them. Businesses would normally be covered under standard commercial coverage for injuries to people on the premises for immunization. Each business should verify its coverage.

Some private businesses, such as grocery stores, may not have a standard commercial policy. Some grocery stores have policies written by surplus carriers which would not cover events such as an immunization drive on the store's premises. In these cases, businesses may need to pay a modest premium for additional coverage.

Liability for Administering Vaccines

The liability exposure for people who administer vaccines is small because of the extensive protections under federal and state laws discussed above. Adverse reactions are often the greatest source of liability concern because of the potential seriousness of the injury and the inability to prevent the random adverse reaction.

If the federal VICP law does not apply because a non-covered vaccine is involved, because negligence is alleged or because the injured person rejects the compensation awarded, the injured person would have to file suit in state court. State laws of the type described above provide significant liability protections. Many provide immunity for people giving immunizations unless the vaccine is administered negligently.

Frequently, immunization programs can be structured to maximize the application of state laws with immunity protections. Many programs probably could be designed so immunizing would be a duty performed under instructions of the state department of health. Many programs could be set up under the auspices of a 501(c)(3) or 501(c)(4) tax-exempt organization, and a state charitable immunities act could provide extensive immunity protections to volunteers. Examples of organizations likely to be exempt under IRS regulation 501(c)(3) are churches, parent-teacher associations, colleges, non-profit hospitals and similar charitable organizations. If a program is set up for a school district, the special protections of the state education code could apply.

Can a practitioner be accountable to a state licensing board if someone is injured by a vaccine? Yes, but no more so than in any other practice setting. The practitioner would be subject to disciplinary action only for failing to comply with minimum acceptable standards of practice, regardless of whether injury occurs. Minimum standards of practice may include:

- Properly assessing the vaccine candidate for vaccine indications and the absence of contraindications;
- Providing appropriate information or education to vaccinees; and
- Responding appropriately to adverse events (eg, summoning emergency personnel, administering emergency treatments).

If a vaccine is administered by a nurse following a physician's order, the physician is generally not liable if the nurse administers the vaccine negligently. In this case, the nurse is acting under the authority of a nursing license. Physicians are not liable for nurses who negligently practice nursing just as they are not liable for laboratories that negligently perform tests.

Physicians can rely on a nurse's license as assurance that the nurse possesses a certain level of competency. Regarding administration of vaccines, physicians can rely on nursing licensure as a reasonable basis for believing a nurse can administer vaccines competently. Of course, if a physician should have recognized that a particular nurse lacks the competency to administer a vaccine, the physician could incur liability. However, the physician would not be liable for the negligence of the nurse, but rather for the physician's negligence in ordering a nurse of questionable competency to give an immunization. Likewise, a physician employing the nurse could incur liability, but that liability would be based on the employer-employee relationship and not on the physician-nurse relationship.

In many states, drug administration is included within the scope of pharmaceutical practice. Presumably the same relationships between physician and pharmacist would operate as in the physician-nurse example in the preceding paragraphs. The physician should be satisfied that the pharmacist can competently administer an immunization (eg, has been trained in proper injection technique). Physicians are not liable for pharmacists who negligently practice pharmacy.

A physician's order for vaccines might take the form of a standing order or protocol. Such a protocol could apply to a patient population, rather than a particular patient. Effectively, the order might say, "Vaccinate all those people who fit ACIP guidelines for immunization." The order may need to describe the patient population, unless a physician can reasonably assume the nurse or pharmacist is knowledgeable about the population. Good clinical practice suggests that standing orders or protocols for vaccines should:

1.) Be signed and dated by the physician;
2.) Identify the vaccines covered by the order;
3.) Indicate that the vaccine candidate should be assessed for vaccine indications and the absence of contraindications;
4.) Indicate that appropriate procedures be in place for responding to reactions to the vaccine; and
5.) Order the administration of the specific medication or category of medication to be administered if a reaction occurs.

A physician does not need to be readily available when the nurse or pharmacist administers the vaccine. Vaccine administration, ordered by a physician, is a nursing or pharmacy act performed under the authority of the nursing or pharmacy license.

Physicians do not need to delegate the administration of vaccines to nurses or pharmacists, because nurses and pharmacists administer the vaccine under the authority of their own licenses. Whether a nurse or pharmacist can delegate the administration of a vaccine to an unlicensed person depends on state professional practice acts.

If delegation of vaccine administration by a licensed person to an unlicensed person is permitted in a state, the licensed professional's liability exposure would be the same as if the licensed professional administered the vaccine. However, the professional also would be liable for the negligence of the unlicensed person. Delegation is like loaning your license, in that the delegated act is performed under the authority of the professional's license. The professional remains accountable for acts done under the authority of his or her license and would be liable to the vaccinee for any injury. The professional also would have the same legal protections available as if he or she had administered the vaccine.

Because of the low liability exposure in administering vaccines, the decision whether to purchase professional liability insurance probably should be based on the actual scope of practice. The decision might be made by the professional or the professional's employer. However, an employer's liability insurance is unlikely to provide coverage outside the employment setting. Having coverage can help ensure the availability of funds to cover an injured person's medical expenses. Check with your employer or local governmental entity or school district to determine what coverage you have. Good Samaritan Acts usually apply only to care rendered in emergencies. They do not appear to apply to immunizations.

Risk Reduction

What are prudent acts to take to reduce liability?

- Attend specialized training in vaccine indications and contraindications;
- Act prudently, within the scope of practice for your profession;
- Mimic the standards and safeguards adopted at your county health clinic;
- Ask good screening questions;
- Obtain informed consent from vaccinees and parents on CDC-endorsed consent forms, with their signatures acknowledging risks and benefits.

It is often prudent to buy liability insurance to protect against unforeseen events not covered.

Failing to Vaccinate

On the other hand, a growing number of lawsuits are being filed for failing to immunize. Negligence can involve failing to adopt an accepted immunization practice. Information collected by the Immunization Action Coalition reveals that most of the known cases were settled out of court. Specific instances involve:

- Failing to offer occupational immunization against measles to a nurse who died of it;
- Failing to immunize against *Haemophilus influenzae* type b in a child who developed Hib meningitis, where the mother reportedly requested the vaccine but the pediatrician was not aware of revised Hib vaccine recommendations;
- Failing to immunize against *Haemophilus influenzae* type b in a child who developed Hib disease and persistent sequelae;
- Three cases of failing to vaccinate the newborn infant of a hepatitis B carrier.

Failing to recognize vulnerability to devastating infection can be as wrongful as failing to detect a problem in an X-ray. Immunize all those in need.

Compensation for Vaccine Injury

If a vaccine injures a child in the US, the family can be compensated under a special federal program. The National Childhood Vaccine Injury Act of 1986 authorized the Vaccine Injury Compensation Program (VICP). The VICP is a no-fault system to indemnify injured children. Indemnification is compensation for loss or damage; to the person who vaccinates, indemnification protects against personal liability.[8,10-18]

Childhood vaccines are exceedingly safe, but they are not perfectly safe. A few vaccinated children are harmed each year by well-intentioned use of a vaccine. Rather than require those children to seek relief through a lawsuit, the VICP eases their burden. In this way, the VICP balances society's need to immunize children and personal risk to individual children.

Vaccines covered by the National Childhood Vaccine Injury Act and VICP include any product containing one or more of these antigens in any form: Diphtheria, tetanus, pertussis, measles, mumps, rubella or poliovirus.

Other vaccines may soon be added to this list (eg, hepatitis B, *Haemophilus influenzae* type b, varicella).

The VICP is administered by the US Court of Federal Claims, the Department of Health & Human Services (HHS), and the Department of Justice (DOJ). A person claiming injury from a vaccine must first file a petition for compensation with the Court. Next, a physician at the HHS Division of Vaccine Injury Compensation compares the petition to criteria for compensation and makes a recommendation in a report filed with the Court by DOJ.

Not all adverse events that follow closely after vaccination are caused by the vaccine. To simplify the issue of whether to blame the vaccine for a given adverse event, events listed in an official Vaccine Injury Table (VIT) are presumed to have been caused by the certain vaccines.

To qualify for compensation, the petitioner must:

- Show that an injury listed in the Vaccine Injury Table occurred within the specified periods,
- Prove that the vaccine caused an injury or
- Prove the vaccine aggravated a pre-existing condition.

The Vaccine Injury Table is a mechanism for defining complex medical conditions. It allows a statutory presumption of causation. Because it is easier to demonstrate a "table injury" than to prove that the vaccine caused a condition, most claims allege a table injury, however, compensation is not awarded if the Court finds that the injury or death was because of a cause unrelated to the vaccine, even if it is a table injury.

The effect of the injury must continue for at least 6 months after vaccine administration. The claim must be filed within 36 months after the first symptom appeared. For claims involving death, the claim must be filed within 24 months of the death and within 48 months after the onset of the injury from which the death occurred. The injured person may file the petition, or a parent, legal guardian or trustee may file for a child or an incapacitated person. In exchange for these simplified proceedings, petitioners cannot file claims for punitive damages or file derivative claims by family members for loss of companionship.

For death-related claims, the total benefit allowed by law is $250,000. In injury claims, the Court fixes the amount of compensation based on the needs of the person and the extent of injury. The award may include past and future nonreimbursable medical, residential, custodial and rehabilitation expenses not otherwise covered by a third-party payer. In addition, the award may include lost earnings, pain and suffering and reasonable attorney fees and costs. While VICP does not provide for punitive damages, its awards are fair and include attorneys' fees. Claims result in an award of damages to the claimant or a determination that the injury is not vaccine-related.

Adjudication

The Court of Federal Claims judges petitions for compensation, with the Secretary of HHS named as respondent. DOJ attorneys represent HHS in hearings before a special master. A special master is an expert attorney appointed by the judges of the Court. The special master considers the medical record, hears testimony, considers other evidence and makes the initial decision on the petition.

Unlike civil liability suits, hearings under the VICP usually last only one or two days. A case found eligible is scheduled for a hearing to assess the amount of compensation. If the case was brought in good faith, most claims found to be noncompensable receive awards for attorney fees and costs. Either party may object to the decision and request review by the Court. Appeals of judgments are heard by the Federal Circuit Court of Appeals.

Awards are paid from the Vaccine Injury Compensation Trust Fund. It is funded by an excise tax on covered vaccines. Authority to collect the excise tax lapsed in 1993, but it was quickly reinstated indefinitely by the US Congress. A floor-stock tax was levied against vaccine users in the interim to make up for lost revenue.

Key documents needed during the VICP process include:

- Documentation of the person's status before the injury;
- Documentation of the vaccination and
- Documentation of the injury and the person's current medical status. Such evidence may be found in prenatal and birth records, clinic notes, growth charts, laboratory and radiology results, hospitalization and emergency records, school records and death records.

The VICP is unusual in being a national liability program. Laws and regulations governing medical malpractice and product liability are generally states' perogatives, but the NCVIA of 1986 and various amendments placed unusual constraints on how vaccine-related liability is judged. Vaccine-injury claims must first be filed with the VICP before civil litigation (eg, malpractice claims) through state tort systems may be pursued. No civil claim can be made against a vaccine manufacturer or vaccine provider (typically in state courts) while a VICP claim is being considered. If a petitioner accepts an award under the VICP, a malpractice claim cannot be brought later in the tort system. Petitioners can reject an award made under VICP and pursue their remedy at tort law, but few do.

Few seek tort relief because their best opportunity is usually the first one. If the neutral VICP special master has already ruled against the case, odds are against other courts reversing judgment. Further, the expense of tort litigation is high and a formidable array of defenses must be overcome.

Healthcare providers cannot be sued while vaccine-injured children and their families are pursuing redress under VICP. Even so, healthcare providers can later be found negligent, such as in giving a vaccination despite an obvious contraindication.

Vaccine Injury Table (VIT) Revisions

An Advisory Commission on Childhood Vaccines meets quarterly to advise the Secretary of HHS on the compensation program and recommend changes in the VIT. The commission is composed of nine private citizens: Three healthcare professionals, three members of the public, and three attorneys.

The 1995 revision of the VIT is a more narrow list of effects that are presumably caused by vaccines compared with the original table. This narrowing is based on several expert panels that reviewed the medical literature and concluded scientifically which adverse events are causally associated with vaccination.[16-18] Please see page 133 for a summary of the VIT table.

For example, if the Institute of Medicine (IOM) found no evidence to support a causal relation of an injury, the Department of Health & Human Services would remove the legal presumption of causation by removing or redefining that injury in the VIT. Nonetheless, acute encephalopathy remains in the table if it occurs within 3 days after vaccination and residual effects persist for 6 months. Chronic arthritis was added to the VIT on the basis of IOM conclusions.[19-21]

Removal of the legal presumption of causation does not preclude a compensation award. Petitioners may still prevail by proving that the vaccine actually caused the specific injury alleged to have occurred.

Synthesis

Contact the VICP at 800-338-2382 or 301-443-6593 for information on how to file a claim, eligibility criteria and documentation required. Write to VICP, Health Resources & Services Administration, Parklawn Building, Room 8A-35, 5600 Fishers Lane, Rockville, MD 20857.

For rules of the Court, call 202-219-9657, or write to Clerk of the US Court of Federal Claims, 717 Madison Place NW, Washington, DC 20005.

Reporting adverse events is also required under the National Childhood Vaccine Injury Act. Procedures for the Vaccine Adverse Event Reporting System (VAERS) are described in chapter 6 on "Immunization Administration."

References

[1] 21 USC 353(b).
[2] Fink JL III, Marquardt KW, Simonsmeier LM. *Pharmacy Law Digest.* St. Louis: Facts and Comparisons, Inc., July 1995.
[3] Archer JD. The FDA does not approve uses of drugs. *JAMA* 1984;252:1054-5.
[4] Nightengale SL. The FDA and drug uses: Reprise. *JAMA* 1985;253;632.
[5] Curran WJ. Influence of the courts of law on biologicals development, regulation, and use. *Bull WHO* 1977;55(Suppl 2):53-65.
[6] Landwirth J. Medical-legal aspects of immunization: Policy and practices. *Pediatr Clin N Amer* 1990;37:771-84.
[7] Texas Department of Health. *The Liability Risk Associated With Immunizing Children.* Austin: State of Texas, 1994.
[8] Grabenstein JD. Compensation for vaccine injury: Balancing society's need and personal risk. *Hosp Pharm* 1995;30:831-2,834-6.
[9] Baker CH, Brennan JM. Legal aspects of hepatitis B immunization programs. *N Engl J Med* 1984;311:684-8.
[10] Centers for Disease Control. National Childhood Vaccine Injury Act: Requirements for permanent vaccination records and for reporting of selected events after vaccination. *MMWR* 1988;37:197-200.
[11] Prins-Stairs JC. The National Childhood Vaccine Injury Act of 1986: Can Congressional intent survive judicial sympathy for the injured. *J Legal Med* 1989;10:703-37.
[12] Clayton EW, Hickson GB. Compensation under the National Childhood Vaccine Injury Act. *J Pediatr* 1990;116:508-13.
[13] Perkins LD. Complying with the National Childhood Vaccine Injury Act. *Am J Hosp Pharm* 1990;47:1260,1262,1266.
[14] Department of Health & Human Services. Commonly asked questions about the National Vaccine Injury Compensation Program. Washington, DC: May 1995.
[15] Department of Health & Human Services. National Vaccine Injury Compensation Program Monthly Status Report. Washington, DC: June 5, 1995.
[16] Department of Health & Human Services. National Vaccine Injury Compensation Program revision of Vaccine Injury Table. *Fed Reg* 1995;60:7678-96.
[17] Evans G. National Childhood Injury Act: Revision of the Vaccine Injury Table. *Pediatrics* 1996;98:1179-81.
[18] Glezen WP. Commentary on the revised Vaccine Injury Table. *Pediatrics* 1996;98:1200-1.
[19] Miller D, Madge N, Diamond J, et al. Pertussis immunization and serious acute neurologic illnesses in children. *Brit Med J* 1993;307:1171-6.
[20] Howson CP, Fineberg HV. Adverse effects following pertussis and rubella vaccines: Summary of a report of the Institute of Medicine. *JAMA* 1992;267:392-6.
[21] Stratton KR, Howe CJ, Johnston RB Jr. Adverse events associated with childhood vaccines other than pertussis and rubella: Summary of a report from the Institute of Medicine. *JAMA* 1994;271:1602-5.

TABLE. Summary of the Vaccine Injury Table (effective March 10, 1995) (from Fed Reg 1995;60-7678-96)

Vaccine or Toxoid	Illness, Disability, Injury or Condition Covered	Time Period for First Symptom or Manifestation of Onset After Vaccine Administration
DTP; P; DT; Td; tetanus toxoid; or in any combination with poliovirus; or any other vaccine containing pertussis bacteria or antigen(s)	A. Anaphylaxis or anaphylactic shock	4 hours
	B. Encephalopathy (or encephalitis)	72 hours
	C. Any sequela (including death) of events above	Not applicable
Measles, mumps, rubella or any vaccine containing these viruses	A. Anaphylaxis or anaphylactic shock	4 hours
	B. Encephalopathy (or encephalitis)	5-15 days
	C. Residual seizure disorder	5-15 days
	D. Any sequela (including death) of events above	Not applicable
Measles-mumps-rubella (MMR), measles-rubella (MR) or rubella vaccines only	A. Chronic arthritis	42 days
	B. Any sequela (including death) of events above	Not applicable
Poliovirus vaccine (other than inactivated poliovirus vaccine)	A. Paralytic poliomyelitis: - in a non-immunodeficient recipient - in an immunodeficient recipient - in a vaccine-associated community case	 30 days 6 months Not applicable
	B. Any acute complication or sequela (including death) of events above	Not applicable
Inactivated poliovirus vaccine (IPV)	A. Anaphylaxis or anaphylactic shock	4 hours
	B. Any acute complication or sequela (including death) of events above	Not applicable

DTP — diphtheria-tetanus-pertussis vaccine
P — pertussis vaccine
DT — diphtheria-tetanus toxoids (pediatric)
Td — tetanus-diphtheria toxoids (adult)

CHAPTER 10

Pharmacy's Role in Immunization Delivery

Pharmacy's Unique Contributions

Millions of Americans are vulnerable to preventable infections but have not been vaccinated.

Pharmacists are becoming more involved in raising immunization rates. They are taking on new roles and taking time out of busy schedules to keep their patients healthy.[1-8]

Many people have to play their part in reducing the death toll from influenza and pneumococcal disease, and pharmacists can be key players in this effort. Pharmacists can advance the public health in three ways: Simple education and advocacy, making room for other professionals to immunize inside their pharmacy or administering the immunizations themselves.

Pharmacy has unique opportunities to protect the nation's health. The unique contributions of pharmacy to immunization delivery are these:[7]

- Identification of specific people who need to be immunized, based on the pharmacy's prescription database and the pharmacist's ability to motivate;[9-10]
- People have unparalleled access to their pharmacist, with extended evening and weekend hours, in all kinds of communities: Urban, suburban, rural. In dozens of rural US counties, there is no physician and the pharmacist is the leading health professional.
- Convenience in or near the vaccinee's own home or office.
- Access to computerized records and modem communications, facilitating the delivery of messages (eg, postcards).
- Pharmacists are a highly trusted source of health information, provided in a setting that is personal and nonthreatening.

An estimated 250 million Americans, walk into pharmacies each week. Because pharmacists are America's most accessible health professional, offering immunizations in pharmacies is a logical way of improving the public's health.

Many groups are interested in increasing childhood immunizations, most obviously the nation's pediatricians. It is not appropriate for pharmacists to disrupt continuity of care and compete with pediatricians who immunize. Many children have no medical home and need a consistent source of vaccine information and advocacy. Pharmacists can help refer people to a physician.

Pharmacists are tremendous partners for the public's health, either as a referral source or an immunization site. More points of immunization delivery are needed to overcome persistent shortfalls in immunization delivery. Pharmacy can be one of the mobilized groups, offering extended hours of access.

Even if many providers in your neighborhood deliver routine childhood vaccines, ask if anyone is taking responsibility for identifying the kids who need influenza and pneumococcal vaccines. Children with heart defects, diabetes, chronic asthma, sickle cell anemia and other chronic diseases need influenza vaccine and pneumococcal vaccine. Pharmacists know these patients' names. They are the users of digoxin, insulin, albuterol, theophylline and similar drugs. More than 5 million children with asthma need influenza and pneumococcal vaccines. Other children in need are those on long-term aspirin therapy. Immunizing them will reduce their risk of Reye's syndrome.[9-11]

Remember, for every child who dies of a vaccine-preventable disease, 400 adults die of vaccine-preventable diseases. Fifty thousand to 80,000 or more people die needlessly every year, mainly from influenza, pneumococcal disease and hepatitis B. Many of these deaths occur despite appropriate antibiotic therapy. Bacterial resistance to antibiotics is becoming alarmingly common.

Pharmacists Make Great Vaccine Advocates

We already know pharmacists are great vaccine advocates:

- 50% to 94% of people are vaccinated based on recommendations of community, hospital and nursing-home consultant pharmacists.[9,11,13-16]
- People were 74% more likely to be vaccinated if prompted by their pharmacist than if unprompted.[11]
- Cues to vaccination are cost-effective: If Medicare paid pharmacists $1.10 to warn high-risk patients and encourage them to be immunized against influenza, Medicare would save $3.55 for each dollar invested.[17] Greater savings would accrue by advocating pneumococcal vaccine simultaneously.

Every pharmacy should warn people who are vulnerable to a preventable infection. The level of involvement can vary with the resources, time and interest of the pharmacist.

The American Pharmaceutical Association (APhA) adopted a policy at its 1996 annual meeting in Nashville calling on pharmacists to take one of three roles in immunization advocacy:[12]

- Pharmacist as educator (setting up motivation centers);
- Pharmacist as facilitator (hosting others who vaccinate);
- Pharmacist as immunizer (protecting vulnerable people).

Recognizing each person's autonomy, more pharmacists do not talk about patient compliance with a prescribed medication regimen. Instead, they refer to adherence, involving the patient in the decision. Similarly, we should move away from talking about prescription (or vaccine) counseling. Instead, think of pharmacists as motivators toward good health behaviors, like immunizations.

Any pharmacy can serve as an immunization information center. This role involves educating patients and families about who needs which vaccine and when and where they are available. In many places, pharmacists can actually give the immunizations that provide the protection. What you do will depend largely on what is needed in your area. Ask your county health director or the immunization division of your state health department what their greatest needs are. Explain your interest in joining the multidisciplinary team that keeps our society healthy.

What Pharmacists Have Accomplished

Vaccine advocacy is part of mainstream community pharmacy practice in several states. In 1994, more than a million doses of influenza vaccine were given in pharmacies from coast to coast.[3,8] APhA is focusing on three areas to accelerate the implementation of care in pharmacies: Diabetes, asthma and immunizations.[21]

Pharmacist protection of adults and children vulnerable to vaccine-preventable infections is a rolling snowball that is gathering momentum. Pharmacy-based vaccine advocacy on a large scale may have begun in Denver, in 1985. More than 400 pharmacies, independents and large chains, joined the Colorado Influenza Alert Campaign. The Colorado program has cultivated one of the best influenza vaccination rates in the country.[3,8,21]

Colorado pharmacies typically gave 200 to 400 vaccine doses at each participating site during each 2- to 8-hour session. Nurses of the Colorado Visiting Nurse Association (VNA) gave the injections, usually near the pharmacy waiting area. As many as 1000 or more doses were given during exceptional sessions. About 30,000 doses of influenza vaccine were given in Denver pharmacies in 1992, and the number rises each year. Newspaper advertising aided the marketing effort.

By the early 1990s, major pharmacy chains in Illinois, such as Osco, were also vaccinating against influenza near pharmacy dispensing areas. Vaccines were offered at least once at each of 250 or more stores. Osco distributed handouts listing sites and dates of availability.[3]

At many of its 1600 pharmacies across the nation, Kmart Pharmacies distributed a handout in every prescription bag for a month during the 1993 influenza season. Captioned "Does this sound like someone in your family?", the sheet went on to describe the health conditions that are indications for influenza vaccine. The handout concluded with an open appeal to take advantage of the health resource represented by their pharmacist. During the following 1994 influenza season, Kmart pharmacies offered influenza vaccine across the country, using contract nurses to deliver the injections.

That year, Walgreens and Apothecary Shoppe sites across the country hosted influenza vaccination sessions for their communities. Many other chains and independent pharmacies did the same. The shots were usually given by professionals from Nurses PRN, VNA or similar contract nursing agencies. Patients were charged a nominal fee for vaccination, often between $5 and $15. Patients eligible for Medicare received immunizations without charge because pharmacists can be reimbursed by Medicare for administering influenza and pneumococcal vaccination. Many people readily paid cash to be vaccinated.[3,10-11,22-25]

A Desire to Do More

In Michigan, a simple approach introduced many pharmacists to the world of vaccines. The Michigan Pharmacists Association (MPA) distributed a three-ring binder with documents explaining immunization delivery to the state's pharmacists. The binder also featured placards and other tools to help pharmacists teach their patients about the importance of immunization.[6]

Researchers at the West Virginia University School of Pharmacy received a $625,000, 5-year grant from the CDC in 1996 to study pharmacies as vaccination sites. In four rural counties of West Virginia, public health nurses immunize children in community pharmacies, both independents and chain outlets, during evenings and weekends. Other educational programs will be conducted and coupons will be tested as incentives.[26-27]

The "Shots Across Texas" childhood immunization initiative featured community and hospital pharmacists in several ways. The Texas Pharmaceutical Association and the Texas Society of Health-system Pharmacists collaborated in distributing suggested activities to their members. One venture involved handouts that asked "Are The Kids Nearest You Fully Vaccinated?" Any off-targeted copies, given to people without children, increase neighborhood awareness by trickling down to neighbors, grandchildren and others. The H-E-B pharmacy chain encouraged its pharmacists to take leadership roles in their communities via its in-store television training network.

Some pharmacists wanted to be more involved in immunizing. In Georgia, Michael R. Reagan, RPh, organized the Georgia Pharmacy Association's (GPhA's) Pharmacy & Immunization Program. Trained as an emergency medical technician, Reagan understood injection techniques well. He developed an immunization certification program for GPhA's June 1994 annual convention. Starting with oranges for practice, more than 70 pharmacists went through a practicum in injection technique.[2,28]

Three weeks later, GPhA organized two teams of volunteers to help give hundreds of doses of tetanus-diphtheria toxoids during a flood emergency near Albany. A year earlier, in April 1993, GPhA members helped with meningococcal vaccine during an outbreak in Douglas County. A lack of training qualified them only to distribute and reconstitute vaccines for that emergency. Reagan believes one of pharmacy's greatest contributions to the public health will come in rural areas. In his practice in Conyers, GA, the medical director of his county health department approved on his immunization-delivery protocol.[29-30]

Pharmacist as Immunizer

The nation's most advanced community pharmacy-based immunization programs are in Washington, Texas and Mississippi. Faculty at the University of Washington, the Washington State Pharmacists Association and the Washington State Board of Pharmacy collaborated to develop a training program for pharmacist-immunizers. The course consisted of 14 hours of videotaped instruction from a widely respected CDC series and a practicum in injection technique. More than 200 pharmacists plus several hundred students have now been trained in the Washington program.[25,31,32]

In a small city in northwest Texas, two pharmacists took some initiative and now the rest of the state is beginning to emulate them. John Bullock and Robby Timberlake, at the Baggett Pharmacy in Levelland, Texas, developed a novel immunization practice to serve their community. They deliver about 25 to 30 immunizations per week, plus 5 to 10 injections of other types. Their model is being imitated in several states. The Texas Department of Health is reportedly considering encouraging similar practices in other parts of Texas.[25,33]

With all this advance work, the APhA decided that the time was right to develop a model educational program for the nation. They wanted it to eventually be replicated in all 50 states. APhA teamed up with the Mississippi Pharmacists Association, Mississippi Board of Pharmacy and the University of Mississippi to sponsor an exhaustive 19-hour program to enable pharmacists to immunize. For 2½ days, 67 pharmacists reviewed disease epidemiology, immunologic pharmacology, persuasion skills, professional resources, ways to overcome barriers, emergency responses and injection technique.

After completing the equivalent of half a semester's work, the Mississippi pharmacists were tested with practical exercises and a 2½-hour comprehensive examination. More than 94% of the pharmacists passed the exam on the first attempt. The curriculum was based on similar CDC training programs, with special emphasis on adult immunization. Adult vaccines were stressed because of the thousands of deaths among adults from vaccine-preventable diseases (eg, influenza, pneumonia, hepatitis B). Despite the difficulties encountered in any pioneering endeavor, almost half the Mississippi trainees were immunizing people within the first 6 weeks after training. In that short amount of time, they had already administered > 5000 immunizations. Repeat training programs in Mississippi and other locations are now being planned.[34-35]

As of April 1997, 18 states permit pharmacists to administer drugs within the scope of the practice of pharmacy: Alabama, California, Georgia, Illinois, Indiana, Iowa, Kentucky, Michigan, Mississippi, Missouri, Nebraska, New Mexico, South Carolina, South Dakota, Tennessee, Texas, Virginia and Washington. Other states are negotiating changes to their professional scope of practice. This information is based on a survey of state pharmaceutical associations. Check with your state's board of pharmacy for the current scope of practice and other regulations related to immunizations.

If your state is not listed above, work with your state pharmaceutical association and board of pharmacy to get your state's pharmacy practice act changed to reflect the new state of the profession. Local chapters of the

American Red Cross teach procedures for adult and child basic cardiac life support/cardiopulmonary resuscitation.

Pharmacists as Vaccine Leaders

Immunization advocacy occurs at the pharmacy counter, at the counseling center, at the patient's bedside, in meeting rooms or anywhere a pharmacist is. In a community pharmacy, the consultation area is often the proper place to give the vaccine doses.

Pharmacies offer major advantages as places to administer immunizations: Access, convenience and knowledge of the individuals most in need.

Vaccines are drugs, and pharmacists are responsible for the most effective use of drugs. If someone suffers a preventable infection, it is a drug-related problem that a pharmacist could have prevented. Greater than 50,000 people die needlessly each year of influenza and pneumococcal disease. Most professionals who have delivered immunizations for years welcome pharmacists to the job, so long as the highest quality standards are observed. These people are easily persuaded by informing them about the preparation and commitment to quality you have made. Explain the specialized training in vaccine indications and contraindications you attended. Act prudently, within your scope of practice. Mimic the standards and safeguards adopted at your county health clinic for vaccine delivery. Ask good screening questions. Obtain informed consent from patients and parents on CDC-endorsed consent forms.

A pharmacist may encounter a professional who is concerned that pharmacists who deliver immunizations will reduce that professional's economic interests in vaccine delivery. Perhaps the best response in this situation is to quote the adage, "A rising tide lifts all boats." There are millions of people at risk who are now unprotected against influenza and pneumococcal disease. There is no need to quarrel over robbing market share from one vaccine provider to another.

Consider the experience of Steven Mostow, MD, long-time chair of the Colorado Influenza Alert Campaign. He helped orchestrate the drug store clinics and public-education media blitz that is a major component of the Campaign. "I spent 20 years trying to convince doctors to give flu shots, and it was a big failure," he said in 1994. "My first year, doctors wrote me nasty letters saying that I was taking their business away and sending it to grocery stores, but they were wrong. It [the campaign] increased overall awareness of immunization. There were 100,000 vaccines [doses] given in doctors' offices when we started, and last year there were 700,000."[3,8,21]

Here are some standards you can adopt for your pharmacy-based immunization program, to convince others of your commitment to quality:

- Focus on the people who die lacking vaccines (eg, influenza, pneumococcal disease, hepatitis B).
- Do not disrupt the medical home. Respect the physician-patient relationship.
- Consult, inform and report as appropriate.
- Do not miss opportunities, in any patient encounter.
- Educate at every opportunity.

- Ask about contraindications, and know the difference between valid and invalid ones.
- Document the vaccinee's informed consent on CDC-endorsed forms.
- Keep perpetual records; give the vaccinee a record.
- Support your health department and local coalitions.
- Be prepared for emergencies.
- Stay up-to-date.

Roles for Community Pharmacists

One of pharmacy's advantages as a site for immunization delivery is its extended hours of availability. Adults like the convenience of being immunized during the evening or on weekends. For the busy parent who cannot take time off from work to get the children to a health clinic, immunizations at a pharmacy can be very attractive. A consumer article advised readers to choose a family pharmacist based on extra services provided, including whether the pharmacy conducted flu shot clinics.[36]

Given America's access to community pharmacists, neighborhood pharmacies are where much of the pharmacy-based immunizations will occur. These are excellent opportunities for people to be educated and motivated to be vaccinated. Any of the roles discussed above can be implemented in your pharmacy.

Roles for Hospital Pharmacists

Similarly, hospital pharmacists can help reduce morbidity and mortality. They can identify people needing vaccines by obtaining immunization histories and providing appropriate recommendations for both inpatient and outpatients.[37]

Hospital pharmacists have a special role to play in assuring that people receive the full preventive benefits of the healthcare system. Advising people about vaccines is an important part of overall patient care and allows the pharmacist to act in a primary care role. Interviewing and motivating people regarding immunizations reflects the preventive aspects of pharmaceutical care.

Pharmacists in hospitals can fulfill each of the three roles in immunization advocacy: Motivation, facilitation or injection. Specific fields include providing drug information, taking vaccine histories as well as drug histories, writing articles in newsletters for staff or patients, providing in-service training for pharmacy, nursing or other personnel, leading pharmacy & therapeutics (P&T) committees, making purchasing decisions, participating on infection-control committees and the like. Pharmacists can advocate vaccines on rounds and at grand rounds. Pharmacists can influence critical pathways, discharge planning and utilization review and quality-improvement programs. Hospital policies on managing needle sticks, possible rabies exposure, wound management in the emergency room, occupational health, pediatric admissions and other topics have implications for vaccine advocacy.

The transformation of America's hospitals into health systems increases the number of places where these pharmacists might encounter people needing vaccines. The physical settings include the hospital, home health-care encounters, long-term care facilities, rehabilitation hospitals, ambulatory care settings and nursing homes.

Roles for Nursing Home Consultants

Many nursing homes do not adequately protect their residents against preventable infectious diseases. Consultant pharmacists can help in this arena, but many have not consistently done so.

Nursing home residents need influenza vaccine; many of them also need pneumococcal vaccine. A survey of Minnesota nursing homes revealed an influenza vaccination rate of 84%,[38] but 35% of homes failed to offer vaccine to residents newly admitted during the influenza immunization season. Whereas 69% of homes had written policies for influenza vaccination, ⅓ had policies for pneumococcal vaccine and only 16% for tetanus-diphtheria (Td). Twelve-month immunization rates were 12% and 3% for these latter two vaccines, respectively. Because the nation has low baseline immunity rates against pneumonia, tetanus and diphtheria, these rates probably leave much of this population vulnerable. Influenza vaccination of employees averaged 33%. Few sites evaluated immunization practices in their quality-assurance program. A Scottish study confirmed the importance of immunizing the staff to prevent influenza mortality of elderly patients.[39] These are situations consultant pharmacists can help improve.

Model Immunization Practices

The following outline offers examples in three levels of immunization advocacy. Within each level, more involved activities for pharmacists are suggested.[11]

Level 1: Pharmacist as Advocate: Operating an Immunization Motivation Center

- Display posters encouraging immunization.
- Wear buttons and do other fun things to celebrate National Infant Immunization Week and National Adult Immunization Awareness Week.
- Distribute handouts ("bag-stuffers") or other messages encouraging immunization.
  - broadcast: to medication recipients
  - narrowcast: to recipients of certain medications, either based on prescription database or when those medications are dispensed.
- Examples:
  - A sample message for influenza and pneumonia vaccines: "Does this sound like anyone in your family?" + vaccine indications.
  - A sample message for children and their families: "Are the children nearest you fully vaccinated?"
- Remind people to bring their vaccine records to every medical visit or hospitalization.
- Prepare drug information with references and information about where and when vaccines are offered locally.
- Answer vaccinee and family questions about informed consent documents.

- Lead the pharmacy and therapeutics committee in rational policies on immunologic drugs.
- Lead the infection-control committee in rational policies on immunologic drugs.
- Lead the institution's quality-improvement program in reducing missed opportunities to boost people's immunity.
- Write articles for newsletters or local newspapers.
- Teach classes to pharmacy, nursing, medical and other staff.
- Teach classes to patients and families.
- Work with hospital or neighborhood efforts to improve vaccination rates.
- Ask your colleagues what they do. Collaborate.

Level 2: Pharmacist as Facilitator: Hosting and Helping Others Who Vaccinate

- Activities listed in Level 1, plus those below.
- Identify people needing vaccines:
  - by occurrence (eg, admissions, discharges, ER visits).
  - by taking immunization histories with drug histories (it's the law in Texas and perhaps other states).
  - by working with utilization review staff and discharge planners to deliver immunizations.
  - by diagnosis (eg, asthma, diabetes, age ≥ 65 years)
  - by building immunizations into treatment plans and critical pathways.
  - by procedure (eg, splenectomy, prescription).
  - by building vaccines into treatment plans and critical pathways.
  - by mass screening (eg, nursing home, students, influenza vaccine).
- Host nurses or public health workers who administer immunizations.

Level 3: Pharmacist as Immunizer: Giving Vaccinations

- Activities listed in Levels 1 and 2, plus those below.
- Obtain credentials to administer vaccines, based on a physician's order.
- As local laws permit, prescribe or order immunizations under a practice protocol.

Unique Legal Issues

Vaccines are prescription drugs. In several states, pharmacists act under practice protocols approved by licensed physicians to initiate immunizations. In other states, pharmacists accept written or verbal prescriptions for immunizations from a physician, then administer the doses under the pharmacy's scope of practice. Mississippi offers a good case in point.

Mississippi's authority for pharmacists to administer drugs is found in the Mississippi Practice Act, Section 73-21-73(aa): "Practice of pharmacy shall mean a healthcare service that includes, but is not limited to, the compounding, dispensing and labeling of drugs or devices; interpreting and evaluating prescriptions; administering and distributing drugs and devices...."

Under regulations of the Mississippi Board of Pharmacy, a pharmacist is considered competent in vaccination procedures by providing evidence of specific training in immunizations. He or she also must be competent to deal with an adverse event (eg, CPR), have a collaborative agreement with a physician or clinic to support the immunization program and to handle emergencies and have a sponsoring physician or county medical director authorizing vaccines.

If vaccines are not on the list of drugs authorized for pharmacists to prescribe in your state or at your institution, work with your board of pharmacy or medical staff. Ask for authority to act under the aegis of the public health, occupational health or community outreach director. Ask the same screening questions as the nurses who administer vaccines at the occupational health clinic or similar sites in your facility. In many of these sites, it is customary for most people to be vaccinated under standing orders without seeing a physician. The physician is called in to consult only on unusual cases. Develop an emergency response plan (eg, epinephrine, CPR, ambulance availability) in case of an anaphylactic reaction.

Other legal issues to consider include assuring adequate liability coverage and complying with the record-keeping requirements of the National Childhood Vaccine Injury Act. Be sure to get individual informed consent from each person or from a parent or legal guardian. Although informed consent may only be required for federally purchased vaccines, it is the prudent thing to do for any immunization. Informed consent is also a means to foster patient and family education. Consent forms are available from health clinics and health departments.

Journey of a 1000 Miles

Being a vaccine advocate and an immunizer is not difficult, but it does require preparation. To get started, learn the issues, gather information, and talk to your county health director or the immunization division of your state health department. Seek pharmacy partners in your county and state pharmacy associations. Expert courses on immunizations are available from several sources. For example, the Centers for Disease Control & Prevention (CDC) offers a 14-hour satellite video training conference several times a year, hosted by state and local health departments. Tapes of these conferences can form the basis of training programs organized by state pharmacy associations. You also might consider volunteering to work with other professionals in county health clinics for a short time.

Some months involve more immunization activities than others. But be sure to make immunizations a year-round concern in your pharmacy. National Infant Immunization Week is always the last week of April. August often focuses on updating children's shots needed to attend school. October is busy with efforts to vaccinate people against influenza, but pneumococcal pneumonia kills people all year long. The same is true for tetanus and hepatitis B.

For the pharmacist getting involved with vaccines, consider these four issues first. Which level will you start with: Level 1–motivator, level 2–facilitator or level 3–immunizer? How much and what kind of additional labor will you need: A technician, a pharmacist, a nurse, or will you direct vaccine traffic to slow times so you can use your current staff? How will you phase in immunizations or one morning or afternoon or evening per week or throughout the week? Some pharmacists handle a vaccine prescription as if it were any other prescription and have people read consent forms and prepare documentation while waiting for earlier prescriptions to be filled.

Remember, pioneering is hard. Ask yourself these questions: Who will be your role model? Who will you call for support or advice? What is your time line? What is a reasonable expectation for vaccine doses in the first month?

Ask your local health department for informed-consent documents for each vaccine. They also can help with obtaining copies of your state's official immunization record. Encourage each of your patients to carry one to every medical visit.

Synthesis

Many people want to increase childhood immunization levels. Pharmacists can help. The public's access to a neighborhood pharmacist can be a big boost to vaccine advocacy.

Fewer clinicians are finding those children who need influenza and pneumococcal vaccines. Pharmacists can influence whether these people live or die. Pharmaceutical care calls for us to prevent drug-related problems. Every death from influenza and pneumococcal pneumonia is a drug-related problem. We encourage you to be a vaccine expert and advocate for your patients. Remember, level 3 is best: Do whatever it takes to become a vaccine administrator in your neighborhood.

References

[1] Grabenstein JD. Counseling your patients about vaccines. *Am Pharm* 1992;32:658-9.

[2] Ukens C. Immunization programs shot in arm for community RPhs. *Drug Topics* 1994;138(Dec 12):39.

[3] Shaffer M. Flu shot fever. *Am Druggist* 1994;209(Jan):30-1,35.

[4] Etzel JV, Brocavich JM. Pharmacist's role in immunization. *US Pharmacist* 1994(Nov);Suppl 3:3-18.

[5] Clepper I. Have needle, will inoculate. *Drug Topics* 1996;140(Jul 8):53-5.

[6] Spring B. Give your patients a shot at better health. *Pharm Today* 1995;1(Aug):10.

[7] Grabenstein JD. Implementing a community immunization program: Pharmacists as vaccine advocates. *J Am Pharmaceut Assoc* 1997;37(Suppl):in press.

[8] Debrovner D. Beyond chicken soup. *Am Druggist* 1994;209(Dec):21-4.

[9] Grabenstein JD, Hayton BD. Pharmacoepidemiologic program for identifying patients in need of vaccination. *Am J Hosp Pharm* 1990;47:1774-81.

[10] Grabenstein JD. *ImmunoFacts: Vaccines & Immunologic Drugs*. St. Louis: Facts and Comparisons, May 1997.

[11] Grabenstein JD, Hartzema AG, Guess HA, et al. Community pharmacists as immunization advocates: A clinical pharmacoepidemiologic experiment. *Internat J Pharm Pract* 1993;2:5-10.

[12] Stover KA. APhA House of Delegates adopts 13 new policies. *J Am Pharm Assoc* 1996;36:394-5.

[13] Spruill WJ, Cooper JW, Taylor WJR. Pharmacist-coordinated pneumonia and influenza vaccination program. *Am J Hosp Pharm* 1982;39:1904-6.

[14] Grabenstein JD, Smith LJ, Carter DW, et al. Comprehensive immunization delivery in conjunction with influenza vaccination. *Arch Intern Med* 1986;146:1189-92.

[15] Morton MR, Spruill WJ, Cooper JW. Pharmacist impact on pneumococcal vaccination rates in long-term-care facilities. *Am J Hosp Pharm* 1988;45:73 (letter).

[16] Grabenstein JD, Smith LJ, Watson RR, et al. Immunization outreach using individual need assessments of adults at an Army hospital. *Public Health Rep* 1990;105:311-6.

[17] Grabenstein JD, Hartzema AG, Guess HA, et al. Community pharmacists as immunization advocates: Cost-effectiveness of a cue to influenza vaccination. *Med Care* 1992;30:503-13.
[18] Hepler CD, Strand LM. Opportunities and responsibilities in pharmaceutical care. *Am J Hosp Pharm* 1990;47:533-43.
[19] Jinks M, Cornely PB, Mayer FS. The pharmacist's role in individual preventive health care. In: Bush PJ, ed. *The Pharmacist Role in Disease Prevention and Health Promotion.* Bethesda, MD: ASHP Research & Education Foundation, 1983.
[20] Anonymous. APhA expands pharmacist immunization initiatives. *Pharm Today* 1996;2(10):23.
[21] Debrovner D. Colorado's crusade. *Am Druggist* 1994;209(Dec):22-3.
[22] Anonymous. Vaccination services present payment opportunities to pharmacists. *Pharmacy Reimbursement & Disease Management Report* 1996;1(Apr):3- 7.
[23] Anonymous. Vaccine administration can improve business and patient health at the same time. *Pharmacy Reimbursement & Disease Management Report* 1996;1(Apr):4.
[24] Lorenz EW, ed. *Coding & Reimbursement Guide for Pharmacists.* Reston, VA: St. Anthony Publishing, Inc., November 1996.
[25] Kritz F. A shot in the arm. *Retail Pharmacy News* 1996(May):1,6.
[26] Anonymous. Study of pharmacists' impact on immunizations. *J Am Pharm Assoc* 1996;36:216.
[27] McCormick EM. Pharmacists join model immunization study. *Pharm Times* 1996;62:48,50,52.
[28] Reagan MR. Creating immunization programs in pharmacies. *Pharm Times* 1995;61(Feb):16,19,22-3.
[29] Powell J. Georgia pharmacists flood Albany with relief. *Georgia Pharmaceut J* 1994;16(9):11-4.
[30] Powell J. Local pharmacists volunteer time and expertise during Douglas County health crisis. *Georgia Pharmaceut J* 1993;15(5):16.
[31] Spring B. Washington state pharmacists train to offer immunizations. *Pharm Today* 1995;1(Aug):10.
[32] Anonymous. How to get Medicare reimbursement for vaccinations. *Pharmacy Reimbursement & Disease Management Report* 1996;1(May):4-7.
[33] American Pharmaceutical Association Foundation. Practice profile: Baggett Pharmacy. *Pharmaceutical Care Profiles* 1996;3(1):5.
[34] Stover KA. Mississippi to train, pay pharmacists to immunize. *Pharm Today* 1996;2(10):1,26.
[35] Anonymous. Immunize Mississippi–It's your best shot. *APhA Academy Reporter* 1996;4(Dec):9.
[36] Hittner P. Is your pharmacist a good doctor? *Better Homes & Gardens* 1996;74(Apr):96,98,100.
[37] American Society of Hospital Pharmacists. ASHP technical assistance bulletin (TAB) on the pharmacist's role in immunization. *Am J Hosp Pharm* 1993;50:501-5.
[38] Nichol KL, Grimm MB, Peterson DC. Immunizations in long-term care facilities: Policies and practice. *J Am Geriatr Soc* 1996;44:349-55.
[39] Potter J, Stott DJ, Roberts MA, et al. Influenza vaccination of health care workers in long-term-care hospitals reduces the mortality of elderly patients. *J Infect Dis* 1997;175:1-6.

CHAPTER 11

Nursing's Role in Immunization Delivery

Nursing's Unique Contributions

The nation's nurses deliver more immunizations than any other health profession. They are accepting new roles and taking time out of busy schedules to keep patients healthy.

Many people have to play their part in reducing the devastating death toll from influenza and pneumococcal disease, but nurses are key players in this effort. Nurses can advance the public health in several ways: Education, advocacy, or administering the immunizations themselves. Nurses can contact and persuade millions of adults and adolescents to receive influenza and pneumococcal vaccines.[1-5]

Even if you are active in delivering routine childhood vaccines, do not forget to locate children who need influenza and pneumococcal vaccines. Children with heart defects, diabetes, chronic asthma, sickle cell anemia and other chronic diseases need influenza and pneumococcal vaccines. More than 5 million children with asthma need influenza and pneumococcal vaccines. Other children in need are those on long-term aspirin therapy. Immunizing them will reduce their risk of Reye's syndrome.[6-7]

Actively monitor the immunization status of all patients who come into your practice. Immunize each patient who needs an immunization but also inquire about the immunization status of a child and siblings who come for appointments. Actively monitor all children who come into your office.

Of those who die from influenza or pneumococcal disease, ½ to ⅔ of them had been hospitalized 5 years preceding their deaths but were not vaccinated.[8-9] Of those who die from influenza or pneumococcal disease, ⅔ saw a physician as an outpatient during the preceding year but were not vaccinated.[9-10]

Nurses as Vaccine Leaders

Immunization advocacy occurs anywhere a nurse is. Whether you practice in a rural, suburban or urban setting, you will want to offer services to meet the greatest needs around you. The same is true whether you are in a community, nursing home or hospital practice.

Nurses are testing new roles as vaccine advocates.[11-15] Nurses in Ontario developed a method of helping child care centers encourage preschool immunizations.[16] Other forms of outreach have also been reported.[13,17-19] Some nurses assist with international travel clinics.[19]

Here are some personal standards you can adopt for your nursing-based immunization program:

- Focus on the people who die lacking vaccines (eg, influenza, pneumococcal disease, hepatitis B);
- Consult, inform and report as appropriate;
- Do not miss vaccination opportunities in any patient encounter;
- Develop preventive care plans as part of the nursing assessment of each patient;[20]
- Educate at every opportunity;
- Ask about contraindications and know the difference between valid and invalid ones;
- Document the vaccinee's informed consent on CDC-endorsed forms;
- Keep perpetual records; give the vaccinee a record;
- Support your health department and local coalitions;
- Be prepared for emergencies;
- Stay up-to-date.

Roles for Hospital Nurses

Similarly, hospital nurses can help reduce morbidity and mortality among people they serve. They can identify people needing vaccines by obtaining immunization histories and providing appropriate recommendations for in- and out-patients.

Hospital nurses have a special role to play in assuring that people receive the full preventive benefits of the healthcare system. Advising people about vaccines is an important part of overall patient care and allows the nurse to act in a primary-care role. Interviewing and motivating people regarding immunizations reflects prevention at its best.

In Asheville, North Carolina, nurses compared two kinds of in-hospital vaccine advocacy against their historical vaccination rates: A nurse practitioner empowered to assess patients' vaccine needs and administer vaccines without an attending physician's signature vs ward nurses suggesting immunizations to physicians ("enhanced usual care").[21] Adult and pediatric patients were assessed. The baseline immunization rate was 3%. For patients allocated to enhanced usual care, 54% had inadequate or no assessment of vaccine needs; only 4% of the patients who needed an immunization received it. All patients on wards with vaccine-managers were evaluated; 47% needed at least one immunization. Of these, 34% were immunized. Patient interactions with the nurse practitioner averaged 15 minutes each.

Nurses in hospitals can fulfill three roles in immunization advocacy: Motivation, facilitation or injection. Specific fields include taking vaccine histories, writing articles in newsletters for staff or patients, providing in-service training, leading pharmacy and therapeutics (P&T) committees, making purchasing decisions and participating on infection-control committees. Nurses can advocate vaccines on rounds. Nurses can influence critical pathways, discharge planning and utilization review and quality-improvement programs. Hospital policies on managing needle sticks, possible rabies exposure, wound management in the emergency room, occupational health, pediatric admissions and other topics have implications for vaccine advocacy.

The transformation of America's hospitals into health-systems increases the number of places where these nurses might encounter people needing vaccines. The physical settings include the hospital, home healthcare visits, long-term care facilities, rehabilitation hospitals, ambulatory care settings and nursing homes.

Roles in Nursing Homes

Many nursing homes do not adequately protect their residents against preventable infectious diseases. Nurses can help in this area.

Nursing home residents need influenza vaccine; many of them also need pneumococcal vaccine. A survey of Minnesota nursing homes revealed an influenza vaccination rate of 84%.[22] Thirty-five percent of homes failed to offer vaccine to residents newly admitted during the influenza immunization season, whereas 69% of homes had written policies for influenza vaccination, ⅓ had policies for pneumococcal vaccine and only 16% for tetanus-diphtheria (Td). Twelve-month immunization rates were 12% and 3% for these latter two vaccines, respectively. Because the nation has low baseline immunity rates against pneumonia, tetanus and diphtheria, these rates probably leave much of this population vulnerable. Influenza vaccination of employees averaged 33%. Few sites evaluated immunization practices in their quality-assurance program. These are situations nurses can help improve.

Nursing Roles in Immunization

- Display posters encouraging immunization.
- Wear buttons and do other fun things to celebrate National Infant Immunization Week and National Adult Immunization Awareness Week.
- Distribute handouts ("bag-stuffers") or other messages encouraging immunization.
  - broadcast to all patients.
  - narrowcast to just high-risk patients, based on nursing diagnosis, care plan or prescriptions.
- Examples:
  - A sample message for influenza and pneumonia vaccines: "Does this sound like anyone in your family?" + vaccine indications.
  - A sample message for children and their families: "Are the children nearest you fully vaccinated?"
- Remind people to bring their vaccine records to every medical visit or hospitalization.
- Answer vaccinee and family questions about informed-consent documents.
- Lead the infection-control committee in rational policies on immunologic drugs.
- Lead the institution's quality-improvement program in reducing missed opportunities to boost people's immunity.
- Write articles for newsletters or local newspapers.
- Teach classes to pharmacy, nursing, medical and other staff.

- Teach classes to patients and families.
- Work with wider hospital or neighborhood efforts to improve vaccination rates.
- Ask your colleagues what they do; collaborate.
- Identify people needing vaccines:
  - by occurrence (eg, admissions, discharges, ER visits).
  - by taking immunization histories with drug histories (it's the law in Texas and perhaps other states).
  - by working with utilization review staff and discharge planners to deliver immunizations.
  - by diagnosis (eg, asthma, diabetes, age ≥ 65 years)
  - by procedure (eg, splenectomy, prescription).
  - by building immunizations into treatment plans and critical pathways.
  - by mass screening (eg, nursing home, students, influenza vaccine).

Unique Legal Issues

Vaccines are prescription drugs. In several states, nurses act under practice protocols approved by physicians to initiate immunizations. In other states, nurses accept written or verbal orders for immunizations from a physician then administer the doses under the nurse's scope of practice.

Other legal issues to consider include assuring adequate liability coverage and complying with the record-keeping requirements of the National Childhood Vaccine Injury Act. Be sure to get individual informed consent from each person, parent or legal guardian. Although informed consent may only be required for federally purchased vaccines, it is the prudent thing to do for any immunization. Informed consent is also a means to foster patient and family education. Consent forms are available from health clinics and health departments. Details appear in other chapters.

Be an Advocate

Being a vaccine advocate and an immunizer is not difficult, but it does require preparation. To get started, learn the issues, gather information, and talk to your county health director or the immunization division of your state health department. Seek nursing partners in your county and state nursing associations. Expert courses on immunizations are available from several sources. For example, the CDC offers a 14-hour satellite video training conference several times a year hosted by state and local health departments. Tapes of these conferences can form the basis of training programs organized by state nursing associations. You also might consider volunteering to work with other professionals in county health clinics for a short time.

Some months involve more immunization activities than others, but be sure to make immunizations a year-round concern in your office or clinic. National Infant Immunization Week occurs in the last full week of April each year. August often focuses on getting children caught up on the shots needed to attend school. October is busy with efforts to vaccinate people against influenza, but pneumococcal pneumonia kills people all year long. The same is true for tetanus and hepatitis B.[7]

Remember, pioneering is hard. For the nurse beginning to get involved with vaccines, consider these issues first. Who will be your role model? Who will you call for support or advice? What is your time line? What is a reasonable expectation for vaccine doses in the first month?

Ask your local health department for informed-consent documents for each vaccine. They also can help with obtaining copies of your state's official immunization record. Encourage your patients to carry one to every medical visit.

Many people want to increase childhood immunization levels. Be sure to help them. Remember that fewer clinicians are finding those children who need influenza and pneumococcal vaccines.

Every death from influenza and pneumococcal pneumonia is a drug-related problem. Be a vaccine expert and advocate for your patients. Do whatever it takes to be a vaccine giver in your neighborhood.[13]

References

[1] Centers for Disease Control & Prevention. Recommended childhood immunization schedule – United States, 1997. *MMWR* 1997;46:35-40.

[2] Advisory Committee on Immunization Practices. Immunization of adolescents. *MMWR* 1996;45(RR-13):1-16.

[3] Centers for Disease Control & Prevention. Assessing adult vaccination status at age 50 years. *MMWR* 1995;44:561-3.

[4] Advisory Committee on Immunization Practices. General recommendations on immunization. *MMWR* 1994;43(RR-1):1-38.

[5] Hutchison BG. Effect of computer-generated nurse/physician reminders on influenza immunization among seniors. *Fam Med* 1989;21:433-7.

[6] Grabenstein JD, Hayton BD. Pharmacoepidemiologic program for identifying patients in need of vaccination. *Am J Hosp Pharm* 1990;47:1774-81.

[7] Grabenstein JD. *ImmunoFacts: Vaccines & Immunologic Drugs.* St. Louis: Facts and Comparisons, May 1997.

[8] Fedson DS. Influenza and pneumococcal immunization strategies for physicians. *Chest* 1987;91:435-43.

[9] Williams WW, Hickson MA, Kane MA, et al. Immunization policies and vaccine coverage among adults: The risk for missed opportunities. *Ann Intern Med* 1988;108:616-25.

[10] Magnussen CR, Valenti WM, Mushlin AI. Pneumococcal vaccine strategies. *Arch Intern Med* 1984;144:1755-7.

[11] Bellig LL. Immunization and the prevention of childhood diseases. *J Ob Gyn Neonatal Nursing* 1995;24:669-77.

[12] Anonymous. Nursing Times guide to immunisation. *Nursing Times* 1996;92(Suppl):12-8.

[13] Huber D. Operation immunize: A nursing opportunity, its success is up to you. *Kansas Nurse* 1993;68(4):4-5.

[14] Pendleton S, Jones M. An immunisation need: The nursing response. *Nursing Standard* 1994;9(Suppl):3-10.

[15] Anonymous. Consensus policy for RN immunization administration. *New Jersey Nurse* 1994;24(9):1.

[16] O'Mara LM, Isaacs S. Evaluation of registered nurses follow-up on the reported immunization status of children attending child care centers. *Can J Public Health* 1993;84:124-7.

[17] Jefferson N, Sleight G, Macfarlane A. Immunisation of children by a nurse without a doctor present. *Brit Med J* 1987;294:423-4.

[18] Ferson MJ, Fitzsimmons G, Christie D, et al. School health nurse interventions to increase immunisation uptake in school entrants. *Public Health* 1995;105:25-9.

[19] Goldsmith J. When wanderlust takes over: Nurse-run foreign travel clinics. *Prof Nurse* 1991;6:609-10,612.

[20] Dickey LL, Griffith HM, Kamerow DB. Put prevention into practice: Implementing preventive care. *J Am Acad Nurse Pract* 1994;6:257-66,errata ....

[21] Landis S, Scarbrough ML. Using a vaccine manager to enhance in-hospital vaccine administration. *J Fam Pract* 1995;41:364-9.

[22] Nichol KL, Grimm MB, Peterson DC. Immunizations in long-term care facilities: Policies and practice. *J Am Geriatr Soc* 1996;44:349-55.

[23] Potter J, Stott DJ, Roberts MA, et al. Influenza vaccination of healthcare workers in long-term-care hospitals reduces the mortality of elderly patients. *J Infect Dis* 1997;175:1-6.

[24] Grabenstein JD, Grabenstein LA. *Pocket ImmunoFacts 1997: Vaccines & Immunologics.* St. Louis: Facts and Comparisons, Inc., 1997.

[25] Kachoyeanos MK, Friedhoff M. Cognitive and behavioral strategies to reduce children's pain. *Maternal/Child Nursing* 1993;18:14-9.

[26] French GM, Painter EC, Coury DL. Blowing away shot pain: A technique for pain management during immunization. *Pediatrics* 1994;93:384-8.

CHAPTER 12

Medicine's Role in Immunization Delivery

Physicians have many key leadership roles to play in immunization advocacy. Their roles constitute a spectrum from education to administration to empowerment of others. This chapter reviews ways physicians can increase immunization levels in their communities.

Maximize Prevention in Your Practice

Build vaccine advocacy into your everyday patient visits. Educate your staff about vaccine indications and contraindications and then empower them vaccinate the people who need it.[1-4]

Even if you are active in delivering routine childhood vaccines, do not forget to locate the children who need influenza and pneumococcal vaccines. Children with heart defects, diabetes, chronic asthma, sickle cell anemia and other chronic diseases need influenza and pneumococcal vaccines. More than 5 million children with asthma need influenza and pneumococcal vaccines. Other children in need are those on long-term aspirin therapy. Immunizing them will reduce their risk of Reye's syndrome.[5-8]

For every child who dies of a vaccine-preventable disease, 400 adults die of vaccine-preventable diseases. Fifty thousand to 80,000 or more people die every year mainly from influenza, pneumococcal disease and hepatitis B. Many of these deaths occur despite appropriate antibiotic therapy. Indeed, bacterial resistance to antibiotics is becoming alarmingly common.[2,5,9-12]

Remove Barriers to Immunization

One of the most important things to do is to adopt either the Standards for Pediatric Immunization Practice or the Standards for Adult Immunization to raise immunization levels in your practice. Change office policies requiring long waits for advance appointments or requiring a comprehensive physical exam as a prerequisite for immunizations.

Eliminate Missed Opportunities

Actively monitor the immunization status of all patients who come into your office. Immunize each patient who needs an immunization, but also inquire about the immunization status of siblings of children who come for appointments. Actively monitoring all children who come into your office will discourage missed opportunities to immunize.[1-3,5-9,11]

Of those who die from influenza or pneumococcal disease, ½ to ⅔ of them had been hospitalized within the preceding 5 years of their deaths but were not vaccinated.[13-14] Of those who die, ⅔ saw a physician as an outpatient during the preceding year but were not vaccinated.[14-15]

Influenza and pneumococcal vaccines have been available for decades, but they are seriously underused. The death rate is rising, even after adjusting for the aging population.[16-19]

Give All Needed Shots

Make sure that your staff gives all the immunizations a person needs at each critical age. Immunization schedules are discussed in chapter 6 on "Vaccine Administration." Some medical providers are hesitant to give more than one or two immunizations at one session. Experts believe that providers may be more hesitant in this regard than parents are. Use every visit to assess and administer needed vaccines. If a patient asks for a flu shot, check to see if he or she needs pneumococcal vaccine.

Know Valid Contraindications

Be sure you and your office staff know the valid contraindications to immunizations. A poster and written summaries are available from your health department. For example, a sore throat or low-grade fever should not prohibit giving an immunization to a child who is due one. Invalid contraindications are addressed in chapter 4 on persuasion.[2-5]

Educate Patients

Put immunization educational posters in your waiting room, give brochures to patients and parents, send reminder cards in the mail for immunization appointments, and show educational videos in your waiting areas. Each of these vaccine advocacy aids is available from your health department. Call for information about posters and brochures. Check the resources annex to this book.

Educate Your Community

Volunteer to be a guest speaker at PTA meetings or child care or child advocacy group meetings on the subject of vaccine-preventable diseases and immunizations. For adult vaccine advocacy, talk to clubs such as Rotary, Lions, Elks or the Knights of Columbus, as well as lung, diabetes or heart association meetings and similar groups.

Encourage Your Colleagues

Remind your colleagues that modern vaccines are effective and cost-effective.[20-21] Vaccination results in 46% less death, 48% to 57% fewer hospitalizations and net savings in direct medical costs of $117 per person vaccinated.[22] A 6:1 cost-savings ratio by vaccinating high-risk elderly in a health-maintenance organization has been found.[23] Research has found that influenza vaccine reduces health resource use by working adults: 25% fewer respiratory illnesses, 43% fewer days of sick leave, 44% fewer physician visits and net savings in direct medical costs of $46 per person vaccinated.[24]

Help Hospitals Participate

Encourage local hospitals to follow the full spirit of the childhood immunization law by actively immunizing every child who is provided outpatient or inpatient services by the hospital. Extend this standard to adult patients as well. Take a leadership role by inserting evaluations of immunization status as part of critical pathways, utilization review and discharge planning. Extend this standard to home healthcare activities.

Help Nursing Homes Participate

Encourage local nursing homes and residential homes to protect residents by actively immunizing every client. Take a leadership role by evaluating immunization status as part of quality improvement.

Not enough nursing-home residents are protected against influenza or pneumococcal disease. A survey of Minnesota nursing homes revealed serious shortfalls in tetanus-diphtheria (Td) immunity, too. Few sites evaluated immunization practices in their quality-assurance program.[25]

Use Free Vaccine

Free vaccine is available for certain children through the Vaccines For Children (VFC) program administered through your state health department. For uninsured or underinsured children in your practice, you can receive free vaccine from the state Department of Health. You may charge a reasonable fee for administration of the free vaccine. Immunizing all children in your practice rather than referring to the public health system will result in more children being immunized.

Medicare reimburses for influenza, pneumococcal and hepatitis B vaccines, for Medicare beneficiaries who have these vaccine indications based on ACIP recommendations. Details about Medicare reimbursement are included in a separate chapter.

Assessment & Feedback

Public and private physicians want their patients to be immunized. A recent study indicates that providers of vaccinations to infants and toddlers may tend to overestimate coverage among children in their practices. National vaccination coverage assessments in 1993 indicate that only 65% to 72% of children were adequately immunized by 2 years of age. A program called "Provider Assessment & Feedback" quantifies vaccination coverage levels, furnishes feedback to the provider and staff and may indicate vaccine delivery problems and solutions.

Provider assessment is the routine review of immunization records to:

- Determine practice/clinic vaccination coverage levels and problems associated with low levels;
- Furnish feedback to provider and staff concerning vaccine delivery practices that may achieve high coverage levels;
- Motivate provider and staff to develop solutions to the problems identified through the assessment;
- Establish incremental goals for improving vaccination practices and coverage; and
- Monitor the impact of improved practices on coverage. CDC computer software is available for entering vaccination record information, determining coverage levels and rapidly generating a standard, explanatory practice assessment report. An example is Clinic Assessment Software Application (CASA).

The information and feedback increases staff awareness and motivates providers to consider actions to increase immunization coverage. Vaccination problems are discussed, goals are established, solutions adopted and implemented, and the impact of policy changes can be measured. Successful experiences in strategies for vaccination delivery can be shared.

Assessing provider coverage motivates provider and staff to seek solutions to problems and introduce vaccine delivery improvements. Improving performance at the provider level translates into higher coverage levels locally, statewide and nationally. Higher vaccination levels will further reduce vaccine-preventable disease morbidity.

Recipients of immunization infrastructure funds must conduct annual performance assessments in public clinics. Funding is provided to each immunization grantee to support public and private provider immunization performance assessment activities. Infrastructure and other grant funds are also available. Funds may be used for computer hardware and for additional assessment staff.

Assessing individual clinic or provider coverage, including furnishing feedback on vaccine delivery and motivating provider and staff to improve practices, contributes markedly to improving vaccination coverage levels. For more information, contact the Program Operations Branch at the CDC's National Immunization Program, 404-639-8209.

References

[1] Centers for Disease Control & Prevention. Recommended childhood immunization schedule – US, 1997. *MMWR* 1997;46:35-40.

[2] American College of Physicians. *Guide for Adult Immunization,* 3rd ed. Philadelphia: American College of Physicians, 1994.

[3] Peter G, ed. *1994 Red Book: Report of the Committee on Infectious Diseases,* 23rd ed. Elk Grove Village, IL: American Academy of Pediatrics, 1994.

[4] Grabenstein JD. *ImmunoFacts: Vaccines & Immunologic Drugs.* St. Louis: Facts and Comparisons, May 1997.

[5] Advisory Committee on Immunization Practices. General recommendations on immunization. *MMWR* 1994;43(RR-1):1-38.

[6] Advisory Committee on Immunization Practices. Pneumococcal polysaccharide vaccine. *MMWR* 1988;37:64-8,73-6.

[7] Advisory Committee on Immunization Practices. Prevention and control of influenza: Recommendations of the Immunization Practices Advisory Committee. *MMWR* 1996;45(RR-5):1-24.

[8] Advisory Committee on Immunization Practices. Immunization of adolescents. *MMWR* 1996;45(RR-13):1-16.

[9] Advisory Committee on Immunization Practices. Update on adult immunization: Recommendations of the Immunization Practices Advisory Committee (ACIP). *MMWR* 1991;40(RR-12):1-94.

[10] Advisory Committee on Immunization Practices. Recommendations of the Advisory Committee on Immunization Practices: Use of vaccines and immune globulins in persons with altered immunocompetence. *MMWR* 1993;42(RR-4):1-18.

[11] National Vaccine Advisory Committee. Adult Immunization. Washington, DC: Government Printing Office, 1994.

[12] Butler JC, Hofmann J, Cetron MS, et al. The continued emergence of drug-resistant Streptococcus pneumoniae in the US: An update from the Centers for Disease Control & Prevention's Pneumococcal Sentinel Surveillance System. *J Infect Dis* 1996;174:986-93.

[13] Fedson DS. Influenza and pneumococcal immunization strategies for physicians. *Chest* 1987;91:435-43.

[14] Williams WW, Hickson MA, Kane MA, et al. Immunization policies and vaccine coverage among adults: The risk for missed opportunities. *Ann Intern Med* 1988;108:616-625.

[15] Magnussen CR, Valenti WM, Mushlin AI. Pneumococcal vaccine strategies. *Arch Intern Med* 1984;144:1755-7.

[16] McBean AM, Babish JD, Prihoda R. The utilization of pneumococcal polysaccharide vaccine among elderly Medicare beneficiaries, 1985 through 1988. *Arch Intern Med* 1991;151:2009-16.

[17] Centers for Disease Control & Prevention. Influenza and pneumococcal vaccination coverage levels among persons aged ≥ 65 years – US, 1973- 1993. *MMWR* 1995;44:506-7,513-5.

[18] Centers for Disease Control & Prevention. Pneumonia and influenza death rates – US, 1979-1994. *MMWR* 1995;44:535-7.

[19] Centers for Disease Control & Prevention. Mortality patterns – US, 1993. *MMWR* 1996;45:161-4.

[20] Sisk JE, Riegelman RK. Cost effectiveness of vaccination against pneumococcal pneumonia. *Ann Intern Med* 1986;104:79-86.

[21] van den Oever R, de Graeve D, Hepp B, et al. Pharmacoeconomics of immunisation: A review. *PharmacoEconomics* 1993;3286-308.

[22] Nichol KL, Margolis KL, Wuorenma J, et al. The efficacy and cost-effectiveness of vaccination against influenza among elderly persons living in the community. *N Engl J Med* 1994;331:778-84.

[23] Mullooly JP, Bennett MD, Hornbrook MC, et al. Influenza vaccination programs for elderly persons: Cost-effectiveness in a health maintenance organization. *Ann Intern Med* 1994;121:947-52.

[24] Nichol KL, Lind A, Margolis KL, et al. The effectiveness of vaccination against influenza in healthy, working adults. *N Engl J Med* 1995;333:889-93.

[25] Nichol KL, Grimm MB, Peterson DC. Immunizations in long-term care facilities: Policies and practice. *J Am Geriatr Soc* 1996;44:349-55.

[26] Potter J, Stott DJ, Roberts MA, et al. Influenza vaccination of health care workers in long-term-care hospitals reduces the mortality of elderly patients. *J Infect Dis* 1997;175:1-6.

CHAPTER 13

Getting Started

This chapter helps you start a program to encourage adults, adolescents and children in your community to be properly immunized. A vaccine-advocacy program protects your patients from preventable infections and increases your personal sense of professional accomplishment. Because of your access to the public, you are uniquely able to advise patients and their families about infection risk and to motivate them to receive vaccines.

Step 1. Gather Local Information About Immunizations

a.) Call your county health clinic (or 1-800-252-9152) to find out:
   1.) Street address and telephone number of clinic: ________________ ____________________________________. (___) _________________
   2.) What vaccines are offered? ________________________________
   3.) Times of vaccine availability:
   Days of the week, hours: ________________________
   Evening hours: _________________________________
   Weekend hours: ________________________________
   4.) Where is the clinic located, in relation to bus routes or parking? ____
   5.) Usual waiting time for immunizations:
   _______ minutes before, _______ minutes after vaccine
   strategy for shortest wait: _________________________
   6. How much do immunizations cost (specify type of patient and vaccine)? ____
   7.) Any other requirements (eg, shot records)? _________________
   8.) Any restrictions on who is eligible for immunization? __________

b.) Call other sources of immunization for similar data (eg, medical centers, walk-in clinics, travel clinics, occupational clinics, physicians, hospitals).

c.) Call your local county or state immunization coordinator to volunteer to work together (or call 1-800-252-9152). See the annexes for more ideas and resources.

Step 2. Prepare Your Practice and Staff

a.) Discuss the need for vaccines, other information and press releases with your professional, technical and clerical colleagues.

b.) Choose a week when you want to conduct your first advocacy effort. You may want to tie the vaccine week with a back-to-school theme, an influenza theme or another eye-catching theme.

c.) Obtain sufficient signs, brochures, posters or other media to deliver your message. Some ideas are included in an annex to this book. High-quality, camera-ready materials may be available from your state immunization coordinator or local immunization coalition.

d.) Send press releases to local daily and weekly newspapers and radio stations. Ask for a reporter to talk to you personally. Check your telephone book for names and addresses of local news media.

Step 3. Implement the Program

a.) Tell your staff your expectations for the program and the important roles they can play.

b.) Answer questions from patients about vaccines using the various lay-language materials provided in this book.

c.) Refer unanswerable questions to your county health department or to the state immunization coordinator. Build a local expert network.

Step 4. Keep Up the Good Work

a.) Immunization advocacy is a year-round need. Even after your program succeeds, you still need to keep people aware of the need for vaccines. Be a vaccine advocate throughout the year.

b.) Encourage age-appropriate immunizations with your expertise. During autumn months, encourage influenza vaccine for all people ≥ 65 years old and adults and children taking certain chronic medications (eg, digoxin, warfarin, insulin, theophylline).

c.) Encourage one dose of pneumococcal vaccine for the people in the preceding paragraph throughout the year.

d.) Communicate with these people via inserts into billing statements or prescription bags or with posters. Work with your county health department and local chapter of the American Lung Association for this purpose.

e.) Use whatever you did this year as a basis for improvement next year.

Community Catalysts

Many communities have formed immunization coalitions of health professionals, business groups and private citizens to increase immunization delivery to vulnerable adults, adolescents and children. Many communities have done this but not nearly enough of them. If you want to be the catalyst in your community to create or enhance an immunization coalition, contact your state immunization coordinator for information about immunization coverage and shortfalls in your state.[1]

Your state immunization program will often have resources available, such as slides, pamphlets, tapes, videos and posters. Educational programs may be available for providers, communities or educators. Some states coordinate speaker's bureaus to inform civic groups.

Key Questions To Help Advocates Get Started[1]

1.) Is there an ongoing public awareness campaign or a plan for providing immunization information to the public? Does the plan include information about the Vaccines For Children (VFC) program? About Medicare reimbursement for influenza and pneumococcal vaccines? Are the materials used culturally appropriate and provided in all relevant languages?
2.) Has a plan been developed for educating providers about missed immunization opportunities and recruiting them to participate in the VFC and Medicare programs?
3.) Has the WIC (Women-Infants-Children) program developed an immunization initiative? What about your state council on aging?
4.) Is full immunization required for entry into child care? Into nursing homes? Are federal Headstart immunization requirements enforced? Are immunization requirements for entry into other early education programs enforced?
5.) Is there a mandate requiring health insurance companies to cover immunizations, and is it enforced?
6.) How much state funding is invested in immunization?
7.) Does your state have a plan for a statewide registry and reminder system? Will it cover children, adolescents and adults? Are there any computerized registry and reminder systems in your state? Is there a state plan for educating public and private providers about the advantages of computerized reminder systems?
8.) How is your state using the CDC grant funds designated for tracking systems?
9.) Survey local public health clinics to find out the hours when immunization services are available, and make sure they are convenient for working families.
10.) Survey child care facilities, early intervention programs, and Headstart programs to find out if they are complying with federal and state immunization requirements. Demand that the state introduce immunization requirements or enforce those that exist.
11.) Encourage your state Medicaid agency to increase reimbursement for administration of vaccines in line with regional fees defined by HHS.

References

[1] Franklin P, Regan C, Lithwick D. *Building a National Immunization System: A Guide to Immunization Services and Resources.* Washington, DC: Children's Defense Fund, 1995.
[2] Gardner P, Schaffner W. Immunization of adults. *N Engl J Med* 1993;328:1252-8.
[3] American College of Physicians. *Guide for Adult Immunization,* 3rd ed. Philadelphia: American College of Physicians, 1994.
[4] Centers for Disease Control & Prevention. Mortality patterns – US, 1993. *MMWR* 1996;45:161-4.
[5] Magnussen CR, Valenti WM, Mushlin AI. Pneumococcal vaccine strategies. *Arch Intern Med* 1984;144:1755-7.
[6] Fedson DS. Influenza and pneumococcal immunization strategies for physicians. *Chest* 1987;91:435-43.
[7] Williams WW, Hickson MA, Kane MA, et al. Immunization policies and vaccine coverage among adults: The risk for missed opportunities. *Ann Intern Med* 1988;108:616-25.
[8] Peter G, ed. *1994 Red Book: Report of the Committee on Infectious Diseases,* 23rd ed. Elk Grove Village, IL: American Academy of Pediatrics, 1994.
[9] Centers for Disease Control & Prevention. Recommended childhood immunization schedule – US, 1997. *MMWR* 1997;46:35-40.

ANNEX A

Advocacy Ideas

Education & Motivation

- Make sure that mothers of newborn children receive immunization information at the bedside; ask your governor to send a letter to every mother welcoming a new citizen to the state, reinforcing the importance of timely immunization and providing information about immunization services.
- Survey employers in the state, including the state government, to find out if the health insurance they provide to their employees covers immunization. Encourage self-insured companies, exempt from state mandates, to cover immunization for their employees voluntarily.
- Hang up posters; wear buttons; distribute handouts. Consider adding auxiliary stickers to prescriptions: "Are you fully immunized?" on bottles of amoxicillin suspension. Put a sticker marked, "You may need influenza or pneumonia vaccines. Ask your physician or pharmacist," on prescriptions for digoxin, theophylline, hypoglycemic medications, etc.
- Lead your infection-control committee in declaring a local observation of National Infant Immunization Week each April or National Adult Immunization Awareness Week each October. Invite the print, radio and television media to a ceremony marking the week to advertise how you protect the public health.
- Conduct educational programs for staff, patients and other groups. Include vaccine information in newsletters. Incorporate immunization routines into diabetic, asthmatic and heart disease clinics. Give talks to local civic, retirement and other groups.
- Devote an issue of your newsletter to explaining the need to protect adults against preventable infections, or review a vaccine-preventable disease every issue or two. Boiler-plate articles for your internal and external publications may be available from your state immunization coordinator.
- Encourage people to retain their vaccine records and take them to all healthcare visits.
- Use your state's immunization record card, computerized immunization profiles, inpatient and outpatient chart entries.
- Order immunization references for your drug information center, such as order pamphlets, videotapes and additional information from the National Foundation for Infectious Diseases, National Coalition for Adult Immunization, Immunization Action Coalition, the Centers for Disease Control & Prevention or your state health department.

Community Collaboration and Leadership

- Join your local immunization coalition. Ask for details at your local health department or chapter of the American Lung Association. Make vaccine advocacy the theme in activities of local civic groups (eg, Rotary, Elks, Lions, veterans groups, parent groups, class projects and church projects).
- Ask colleagues in your home town what they are doing, and possibly collaborate. Ask local medical, pharmacy or nursing associations to discuss vaccine advocacy at future meetings.
- Offer to help the county with automated vaccine patient profiling.
- Host a mobile van providing immunizations.
- Encourage local businesses, civic organizations and congregations to become involved. Ask for a donation of child-care space for siblings of children getting shots, services such as printing or radio air time or gifts for families who get their children immunized. Include immunization information in religious notices, organization mailings and on the back of utility bills and bank or credit card statements when possible.
- Suggest that local health department clinics and FQHCs develop a friendly rivalry comparing immunization rates at each site. Every 3 months, or the staff of the clinic with the lowest rate could host a small party, picnic or barbecue for the staff of the other clinics.
- Encourage the state health department or a local civic organization to recognize providers who have achieved high immunization rates among their preschoolers. Gold, silver or bronze plaques could be awarded annually for reaching targeted immunization rates.

Stop Missed Opportunities

- Influence institutional policies at hospitals, nursing homes, schools, etc. Codify your vaccine-use policies, following national guidelines:
  - hepatitis B (pre-exposure and needle-stick)
  - rabies prophylaxis (to prevent overvaccination)
  - diphtheria-tetanus-pertussis (DTP) to diphtheria-tetanus (DT) conversion in pediatrics (strict criteria, to maximize pertussis prophylaxis)
  - wound management
  - risk-management policies (do not discharge a susceptible, vulnerable child into the community)
  - infection-control policies (do not let a disease outbreak start among your cluster of children).
  - occupational-health policies (do not let a staff member transmit measles to a patient)
    - Lead your pharmacy & therapeutics (P&T) committee in recommending standing orders for influenza and pneumococcal vaccine for patients receiving appropriate medications for appropriate clinical pathways or discharge diagnoses.
    - Collaborate with your utilization review and discharge planning colleagues to encourage immunizations to adults and children in need. Build immunization advocacy into continuous quality-improvement (CQI) activities or drug-use evaluation (DUE) programs.

- For every admission with a vaccine-indicating diagnosis, recommend influenza and pneumococcal vaccination upon discharge. Use adhesive notes, index cards, letters, chart notes, etc. Send a generic inquiry to the attending physician, and make it hard to overlook the immunization status of the patient.
- For every discharge, send a message that says something like: "We want to keep you and your family healthy. Is everybody adequately vaccinated?" Offer to help adults and children find out what vaccines they need.
- Vaccinate people at risk just before or after discharge.
- Start screening for vaccine needs by medication use; send an individualized, preprinted message recommending vaccination.
- Start taking immunization histories on everybody. Add this information to computerized patient profiles so that dates for booster doses can be generated. In Texas, it is the law that all medical providers must assess the immunization status of all patients 0 to 18 years old at every visit. If vaccine needs are identified, the provider must either give the immunization or actively refer the patient to an immunization site.
- Encourage your own parents and older relatives to be vaccinated.

Grass-Roots Coalitions

If you are building your own grass-roots immunization-advocacy coalition, consider two dated but thorough manuals:

National League for Nursing. *Guidelines for Volunteer Participation in Childhood Immunization Programs.* New York: NLN, 1980.

National League for Nursing. *Protect Every Child: Childhood Immunization Community Action Kit.* New York: NLN, 1978.

The two manuals cover topics as diverse as marketing and publicity plans, recognition of volunteers, volunteer supervision, gaining co-sponsors, steering committee agenda, school surveys and more.

Ten Things to Do First

Product Oriented:

1.) Delete tetanus toxoid from institutional formularies in favor of tetanus-diphtheria toxoids (adult strength, Td) to sustain diphtheria immunity in the population.

2.) Trivalent measles-mumps-rubella (MMR) vaccine should be favored over single or double-antigen formulations to boost immunity against each of the three diseases. Requests for single- or double-antigen vaccines should be changed to trivalent MMR, in consultation with the prescriber, as frequently as possible. Promote delivery of the second MMR dose.

3.) Tuberculin PPD should be favored over old tuberculin (OT), because PPD is more sensitive and specific than OT, producing fewer false-negative and fewer false-positive reactions.

Information Oriented:

4.) Order references for a drug information center.

5.) Codify vaccine-use policies: Hepatitis B (preexposure and needle-stick), rabies (to prevent overuse), DTP to DT switch, wound management (tetanus-diphtheria, rather than tetanus toxoid alone).
6.) Plan education programs for pharmacy staff, nurses, physicians, patients and others. Use classes, newsletters, memos and P&T meetings.

Patient Oriented:

7.) Start screening for vaccine needs by drug use (eg, digoxin, theophylline, insulin and oral hypoglycemics). Use adhesive notes, index cards, letters, chart notes, etc.
8.) Increase use of influenza and pneumococcal vaccines by staff and patients.
9.) Start keeping vaccine profiles and taking vaccine histories.
10.) Encourage your own parents and older relatives to be vaccinated against influenza and pneumococcal pneumonia.

ANNEX B

Resources

Print Resources

The primary sources of America's vaccine policies are written by the CDC's Advisory Committee on Immunization Practices (ACIP) and by the Committee on Infectious Diseases of the American Academy of Pediatrics (AAP). Other major policy-setting groups include the American College of Physicians and the American Academy of Family Practitioners.

ACIP recommendations are published periodically in the *Morbidity & Mortality Weekly Report.* The *MMWR* can be accessed by traditional subscription or via the Internet at http://www.cdc.gov/epo/mmwr/mmwr.html/. Vaccine information may either be in the main document or in the "Recommendations & Reports" (R&R) supplements. A subscription to the print edition costs $65 per year (617-893-3800).

The 24th edition of the American Academy of Pediatrics' *Report of the Committee on Infectious Diseases,* better known as the "Red Book," will be published in 1997 (telephone 708-228-5005).

The American College of Physicians published the third edition of *Guide for Adult Immunization* in 1994 (800-523-1546).

Facts and Comparisons updates its reference book, *ImmunoFacts: Vaccines & Immunologic Drugs,* and publishes the *Booster Shots* newsletter (800-223-0554). *Pocket ImmunoFacts: Vaccines & Immunologics* is published annually.

A variety of patient-oriented posters and pamphlets are available from the major vaccine manufacturers and private advocacy groups. Telephone numbers for their offices are listed in the following pages.

The National Immunization Program (NIP) at the CDC conducts Satellite Video Conferences. The program on "Epidemiology and Prevention of Vaccine- Preventable Diseases" is conducted in four weekly modules, totaling 14 hours of continuing education experience. Other topics are also broadcast, such as "Update on Adult Immunization," "Vaccines for International Travel" and "When to Immunize, When to Wait," and others. Contact your state immunization program manager, public health adviser, or project director for information on registration and downlink locations. All sessions start at noon EST. Registrants receive a copy of NIP's textbook, *The Epidemiology and Prevention of Vaccine-Preventable Diseases.*

National Immunization Observations	
National Infant Immunization Week (last full week of April)	National Adult Immunization Week (second week of October)
April 20-26, 1997	October 12-18, 1997
April 19-25, 1998	October 11-17, 1998
April 18-24, 1999	October 10-16, 1999

State Immunization Program Managers

Call your state's immunization, hepatitis and refugee coordinators, and get to know your governmental resource people. They often have patient and provider educational materials, including posters, brochures and videos. Call them to register for CDC's immunization conferences that are broadcast by satellite. They also may help you audit your clinic's immunization rates or help you develop immunization tracking systems.

Alabama	334-242-5023	334-613-5325	
Alaska	907-269-8000		
Arizona	602-230-5852	602-506-6657	
Arkansas	501-661-2784	501-661-2053	
California	510-540-2065	510-540-2879	916-323-6614
Los Angeles	213-240-7714	213-744-6191	
Colorado	303-692-2669	303-692-2668	303-692-2678
Connecticut	860-509-7929	860-509-7994	860-509-7723
Delaware	302-739-4746		
District of Columbia	202-576-7130	202-645-5561	202-727-2317
Florida	904-487-2755	904-488-3435	
Georgia	404-657-3158	404-657-2552	
Hawaii	808-973-9640	808-973-9644	808-586-4616
Idaho	208-334-5942	208-334-5638	208-799-3100
Illinois	217-785-1455		
Chicago	312-746-5380	312-814-1884	312-744-2144
Indiana	317-383-6435	317-383-6586	317-383-6420
Iowa	515-281-4917	515-242-5149	
Kansas	913-296-5593	913-296-6512	913-296-4022
Kentucky	502-564-4478	502-781-8039	
Louisiana	504-483-1900	318-345-1700	504-568-5275
Maine	207-287-3746	207-287-6730	207-287-3748
Maryland	410-767-6679	410-767-6672	410-767-5067
Baltimore	410-545-3050	410-767-6665	
Massachusetts	617-983-6834	617-983-6800	617-983-6590
Michigan	517-335-8159	517-335-9423	517-335-8533
Detroit	313-256-1873	313-876-0432	
Minnesota	612-623-5569	612-623-5372	612-623-5693
Mississippi	601-960-7751		
Missouri	573-751-6133	573-751-6122	
Montana	406-444-3624	406-444-2920	406-523-4750

Nebraska	402-471-2937	402-471-0301	
Douglas	402-444-3771		
Nevada	702-687-4800		
Clark	702-383-1494		
Washoe	702-328-3653		
New Hampshire	603-271-4482	603-271-4634	603-271-4494
New Jersey	609-588-7512	609-588-7500	
New Mexico	505-827-2369/2366	505-827-2369	505-827-2495
New York	518-473-4437	518-474-1944	518-474-4845
New York City	212-285-4610/4617	718-520-8245	212-566-7873
North Carolina	919-733-7752	919-715-6760	919-715-3119
North Dakota	701-328-4556	701-328-4550	
Ohio	614-466-4643	614-466-0247	614-644-8162
Oklahoma	405-271-4073		
Oregon	503-731-4020	503-731-4136	503-248-3149
Pennsylvania	717-787-5681	717-787-3350	
Philadelphia	215-875-5649	215-685-6748	215-685-6792
Rhode Island	401-277-1185 x188	401-277-1185 x176	401-277-2312
South Carolina	803-737-4160		
South Dakota	605-773-3737		
Tennessee	615-741-7343	615-532-2695	
Texas	512-458-7284	512-458-7494	
Houston	713-794-9267	713-798-0812	713-439-6180
San Antonio	210-207-8794	210-207-8793	
Utah	801-538-9450	801-538-6191	
Vermont	802-863-7638	802-863-7639	802-863-7333
Virginia	804-786-6246	804-786-6247	804-786-6251
Washington	360-753-3495	206-644-3642	360-705-6770
West Virginia	304-558-2188		
Wisconsin	608-266-1339	608-266-8621	608-267-9000
Wyoming	307-777-7952	307-777-7466	
Territories			
American Samoa	011-684-633-4606	011-684-666-1222	
Federated States of Micronesia	011-691-320-2619		
Guam	011-671-734-7135		
Mariana Islands	011-670-234-8950 x2001		
Republic of the Marshall Islands	011-692-625-3480		
Republic of Palau	011-680-488-1757	011-680-488-2813	
Puerto Rico	809-274-5634	809-721-2000	
Virgin Islands	809-776-8311 x270	809-776-8311 x2148	

Partners in Immunization Advocacy

- American Academy of Pediatrics (AAP), 141 Northwest Point Boulevard, PO Box 927, Elk Grove Village, IL 60009-0927; 708-228-5005; 800-433-9016. http://www.aap.org/.
- American College of Physicians (ACP), Independence Mall West, Sixth Street, Philadelphia, PA 19106-1572; 800-523-1546, 215-351-2600.
- American Diabetes Association (ADA), 1660 Duke Street, PO Box 25757, Alexandria, VA 22313; 800-227-6776, 212-683-7444. For local chapters, consult your telephone book. http:/www.diabetes.org/.
- American Heart Association (AHA), 7320 Greenville Avenue, Dallas, TX 75231; 214-706-1340. For local chapters, consult your telephone book. http://www.amhrt.org/.
- American Lung Association (ALA), 1740 Broadway, New York, NY 10019-4374; 212-315-8700. For local chapters, call 800-LUNG-USA or consult your telephone book.
- American Pharmaceutical Association (APhA), 2215 Constitution Avenue NW, Washington, DC 20037-2981; 800-237-2742, 202-628-4410.
- Canadian National Advisory Committee on Immunization (NACI), c/o Laboratory Center for Disease Control, Ottawa, Ontario K1A 0L2, Canada; 613-957-0841, 613-957-0318, fax updates: 613-941-3900, other fax: 613-957-2990. Health Information for Canadian Travelers: http://www.hpb1.hwc.ca:8500/trav_inf.html/.
- Centers for Disease Control & Prevention (CDC, sic), 1600 Clifton Road NE, Atlanta, GA 30333 (Pamphlets, posters, guidance, sample consent forms, emphasizing sexually transmitted diseases, immunizations, and tuberculosis control):

Consumer Information, English	800-232-2522
Consumer Information, Spanish	800-232-0233
Disease Hotline	404-332-4555
Fax-back Information Service	404-332-4565
Fax document requests to:	404-639-8614
Hepatitis Hotline	404-332-4555
Immunization Division	404-639-1857/1880
International Travel Hotline	404-332-4559
National Immunization Program (professional information)	800-CDC-SHOT
Technical Information Services Branch	404-639-1838
Voice Information System	404-332-4555

  Internet: http://www.cdc.gov or www.cdc.gov/diseases/immun.html/ or www.cdc.gov/travel/travelmap.html/ For MMWR: www.cdc.gov/epo/mmwr/mmwr.html/
  National Immunization Program: nipinfonip1.em.cdc.gov
- Children's Action Network, 1010 Wisconsin Avenue NW, Washington, DC 20007, 202-338-8700.
- Children's Defense Fund, 25 E Street NW, Washington, DC 20001, 202-628-8787; 202-662-3652.
- Every Child by Two, 705 8th Street SE, Washington, DC 20003, 202-544-0808, 202-651-7226.

- Food & Drug Administration (FDA), 5600 Fishers Lane, Rockville, MD 20857; http://www.fda.gov/

Office of Consumer Affairs	301-443-3170
Public Information	301-443-1544
Vaccine Adverse Events Reporting System	800-822-7967, 301-295-8425

- Government Printing Office, Superintendent of Documents, Washington, DC 20752; 202-783-3238 (For PHS Form 731, the "yellow shot record," and Health Information for International Travel). http://www.access.gpo.gov/
- Health Care Financing Administration, US Department of Health and Human Services, HHH Building, Room 307H, 200 Independence Avenue SW, Washington, DC 20201.
- Health Departments, State and Local: consult your telephone book.
- Immunization Action Coalition, 1573 Selby Avenue, St. Paul, MN 55104; 612-647- 9009, fax 612-647-9131. http://www.immunize.org (*Needle Tips, Hepatitis B Coalition News,* and other resources).
- Merck Vaccine Division of Merck and Co., West Point, PA 19436; 215-661-5000, 800-672-6372, 800-NSC-MERCK (a source of news-media kits, reminder cards, profile cards, stickers, other forms and pamphlets). http://www.merck.com:80/mvd/home.html/.
- National Coalition for Adult Immunization (NCAI), 4733 Bethesda Avenue, Suite 750, Bethesda, MD 20814-5228; 301-656-0003, fax 301-907-0878. http://www.medscape.com/NCAI/.
- National Foundation for Infectious Diseases (NFID), 4733 Bethesda Avenue, Suite 750, Bethesda, MD 20814-5228; 301-656-0003, fax 301-907-0878 (posters, pamphlets). http://www.medscape.com/NFID/.
- National Institute on Aging, PO Box 8057, Gaithersburg, MD 20898-8057; 800-222-2225; 800-222-4225 (TTY).
- National Vaccine Injury Compensation Program, Health Resources & Services Administration, 6001 Montrose Road, Room 702, Rockville, MD 20852; 800-338-2382, 301-443-6593.
- National Vaccine Program Office, 56 Fishers Lane, Rockwall II Building, Rockville, MD 20857; 301-594-6350.
- Office of Disease Prevention & Health Promotion, US Public Health Service, 330 C Street SW, Mary E. Switzer Building, Room 2132, Washington, DC 20201; 202-472-5660. http://odphp.oash.dhhs.gov/ [sic].
- Pasteur-Mérieux-Connaught, Route 611, PO Box 187, Swiftwater, PA 18370-0187; 800-VACCINE, 800-822-2463, 800-VACCINE, 717-839-7189, fax 717-839-0940. Protection Plus Kit. http://www.connaught.com/.
- Rotary International, One Rotary Center, 1560 Sherman Avenue, Evanston, IL 60201, 708-866-3000.
- SmithKline Beecham Pharmaceuticals, 1 Franklin Plaza, Box 7929, Philadelphia, PA 19101; 800-999-9384, 800-366-8900, 800-877-1158, 215-751-4000, 215-751-5231, fax 215-751-3400. http://www.sb.com.
- World Health Organization (WHO), Global Programme on Vaccines, CH-1211 Geneva 27, Switzerland; 41-791-21-11.

Regional Office for the Americas: Pan American Sanitary Bureau, 525 Twenty-third Street NW, Washington, DC 20037; 202-861-3200. Publications Center: 49 Sheridan Avenue, Albany, NY 12210; 518-436-9686. http://www.who.ch/

- Wyeth-Lederle Vaccines & Pediatrics, PO Box 8299, Philadelphia, PA 19101-1245; 800-321-2304, 215-688-4400, 215-971-5400; Wasp & Biddle Streets, PO Box 304, Marietta, PA 17547, 717-426-1941, 800-FLU-SHIELD.

Additional Contacts

The following organizations offer a variety of resources, including newsletters, brochures, fact sheets, posters and informational data bases.

All Kids Count	404-687-5615
American Liver Foundation	800-223-0179
COSSHMO (National Coalition of Hispanic Health Organizations	800-232-0233
Hepatitis B Coalition	612-647-9009
Hepatitis B Foundation	215-884-8786
Hepatitis Foundation International	800-891-0707
Immunization Education and Action Committee	202-863-2414
National Council of Black Churches	202-371-1091
National Council of La Raza	301-604-7983
National Digestive Diseases Information Clearinghouse	301-654-3810
National Hispanic Immunization Hotline	800-232-0233
National Immunization Information Hotline	800-232-2522 (English) 800-232-0233 (Spanish)
National Institute on Aging	800-222-2225
Parke-Davis & Co.	800-223-0432
Vaccine Adverse Events Reporting System	800-822-7967, 301-295-8425
Vaccine Injury Compensation Program	800-338-2382, 301-443-6593
Vacunas desde la cuna (Hispanic immunization hotline)	800-232-0233
Visiting Nurses Association	800-426-2547

Product Catalogs

Several organizations offer impressive catalogs of resources for patient teaching and other immunization advocacy activities:

- Immunization Action Coalition and Hepatitis B Coalition, 1573 Selby Avenue, St. Paul, MN 55104, 612-647-9009, fax 612-647-9131. E-mail: editor@immunize.org. Internet: http://www.immunize.org.
- National Coalition for Adult Immunization and National Foundation for Infectious Diseases, 4733 Bethesda Avenue, Suite 750, Bethesda, MD 20814-5228; 301-656-0003, fax 301-907-0878. http://www.medscape.com/NCAI/ or http://www.medscape.com/NFID/. E-mail: nfid@aol.com.
- CDC has many excellent resources including ACIP statements, videos, posters and brochures. For a list of what you can order, fax your request for the "CDC/NIP Resource Request List" to 404-639-8828. The list will be mailed to you.

ANNEX C

Vaccine Adverse Event Reporting System (VAERS) and MedWatch

Despite all precautions to the contrary, adverse events associated with immunization occur rarely. To monitor the safety of vaccines, the Food & Drug Administration (FDA) and the Centers for Disease Control & Prevention (CDC) rely on health professionals to report adverse events. Reporting certain events is required by federal law.[1,2]

This annex focuses on the Vaccine Adverse Events Reporting System (VAERS). Other problem hotlines exist, including FDA's MedWatch and the Drug Product Problem Reporting System, operated by FDA and the US Pharmacopeial Convention (USP).[3,4] The Medication Error Reporting System is operated by the Institute for Safe Medication Practices and USP.

Adverse Events After Immunization

VAERS originated with the National Childhood Vaccine Injury Act (NCVIA) of 1986. FDA and CDC operate and maintain VAERS through a contractor. VAERS began operating in November 1990, replacing separate adverse-event reporting systems at CDC and FDA. FDA Form 3500, the MedWatch form, continues to be used to report adverse events for other drugs, including antibody products and other immunologic drugs.[2,5-8]

VAERS accepts reports of any adverse event related to a vaccine licensed in the US. At present, there are over 40,000 reports recorded in the VAERS database. Upon receipt, VAERS reports are checked for missing information and entries out of the normal range of values for each field. All reports are assigned a unique number and acknowledged.

Reports to VAERS come from a variety of sources:

- Manufacturers (40%);
- State health coordinators and public-sector vaccine providers (35%);
- Private-sector vaccine providers (23%); and
- Parents, guardians and other sources (2%), including vaccinees themselves, other relatives, neighbors and friends.

VAERS personnel then enter the report into a database. At 60 days and again at 1 year after receiving a report of a serious event, they send letters to the reporter for an update on the status of the patient.

VAERS is a passive surveillance system, reports are initiated by the primary observer of the adverse event. Because of its passive nature, VAERS is subject to limitations common to all passive surveillance:[9]

- Underreporting of events;
- Variable accuracy and completeness of reporting; and
- Lack of denominator data (the number of vaccine doses actually given);

An important event may be caused by a vaccine, but if a professional does not report it, the healthcare system never learns from the event that affected the patient. Because the extent of underreporting is large and generally unknown, VAERS cannot be used to estimate the true incidence of an adverse event. This makes evaluation of vaccine-related adverse events difficult.

It is very important to report serious events. Healthcare workers are more likely to report side effects that have already been associated with a given drug. It is important to report to VAERS all serious events that might be associated with a vaccine, whether or not causation by the vaccine is considered probable.

Underreporting varies from one adverse event to another. Because the extent of reporting ranges from < 1% for some events and perhaps up to 50% for others, accurate calculation of adverse-event rates is not possible at present. If underreporting by clinicians were closer to zero, the degree of uncertainty would be greatly reduced.

Members of the public and even some health professionals tend to think of temporal association as proof of causation. As a result, one of the strongest factors for submission of a report to VAERS is a short interval between vaccination and onset of event. Reports to VAERS are frequently evidence of temporal association only. We refer to "adverse events," rather than "adverse reactions," to reflect objectivity before reaching a judgment of causal association.

Batch Surveillance

In addition to using the VAERS database to track reported adverse events, FDA performs surveillance of individual vaccine batches or lots. By using confidential vaccine lot data voluntarily provided by vaccine manufacturers, FDA calculates reporting rates associated with specific production lots of vaccine. It is theoretically possible that faulty manufacture or some other factor might lead a lot of vaccine to have a higher reporting rate than other lots of the same vaccine from the same manufacturer. As one of its regulatory responsibilities, the FDA continually looks for such problem lots and decides whether action is needed to protect the public.[1-2]

Reporting rates result form dividing the number of reports about a vaccine lot by the lot size in doses. Reporting rates are not incidence rates and cannot be used to calculate true rates of adverse events. Lacking such incidence information, the FDA uses reporting rates to look for problem lots. Just as individual reports might indicate either coincidence or causality, vaccine lots may be associated with high rates either chance or true problems. The FDA has developed procedures to assess reporting rates. They help evaluate whether a lot may be associated with a high reporting rate by chance or whether the reporting rate is so high that chance fluctuations are unlikely to be the explanation. Medical evaluations of the types and patterns of adverse events associated with the lot also contribute to these decisions.

Public Information

Summaries of the VAERS database are available to the public via the National Technical Information Service (703-487-4650). Data available in this way include most of the data describing the adverse events reported. Excluded are confidential identifiers, especially names and locations of patients, and proprietary information from manufacturers.[1-2]

Some private-sector groups sell lists of VAERS reports associated with specific vaccine lot numbers. However, data presented in this way is of little value to the public, because lists of lots tell nothing about rates of events observed or expected. Many VAERS reports are not causally related to vaccination. Moreover, the number of reports received in association with an individual lot depends mostly on the size of the lot and the amount of time that it has been in use.

Members of the public might want to know which vaccine lots have few associated adverse-event reports. Unfortunately, the lots most likely to have the fewest reports are those that have been in use for the shortest time. Such lots have not been in use long enough to be associated with many adverse-event reports.

VAERS Utility

Although there are many limitations to passive surveillance such as VAERS, this system can be and is being used for the following purposes:[1-2]

- To detect rare, previously unrecognized, reactions to vaccines;
- To detect increases in frequencies of known reactions to vaccines;
- To detect preexisting or concomitant conditions that may promote reactions to vaccines; and
- To detect particular vaccine lots with unusual frequencies or types of reported events.

VAERS acts as a sentinel, watching for signals that will advance the safety of immunization policies. No lot of vaccine has been associated with numbers or kinds of adverse events likely to be attributable to biological characteristics of the particular lot. Therefore, no lot of vaccine has yet been recalled because of the FDA's lot tracking procedures.

How to Report to VAERS

Submit vaccine adverse-event reports on Form VAERS-1. Copies of the VAERS-1 report form and help in completing it are available by calling 800-822-7967. Completed forms can be faxed to 301-309-6495, or mail VAERS reports to VAERS, PO Box 1100, Rockville, MD 20849-1100. The capacity for public access to some VAERS data is being developed as is electronic submission.

Medwatch

FDA's MedWatch program is used to report adverse events and product problems with human drug products, biological products, medical devices, special nutritional products and other products regulated by FDA. MedWatch is intended to simplify and standardize previous reporting systems, producing a faster and more effective surveillance system.[4] Completed forms can be mailed to FDA, faxed to 800-FDA-0178 or sent by modem to 800-FDA-7737. FDA is most interested in hearing about cases in which a medical product was associated with a serious outcome, such as death, a life-threatening condition, initial or prolonged hospitalization, a disability or a congenital anomaly. It is particularly interested in product reports on the market for < 3 years, because that is when most critical problems are discovered.

Actions taken by FDA after analysis of safety data can include "Dear Health Professional" letters, product labeling changes (eg, boxed warnings), manufacturer-sponsored postmarketing studies and product withdrawals. FDA experience with silicone breast implants, temafloxacin and use of angiotensin-converting enzyme (ACE) inhibitors during pregnancy highlight the vital role that reports from health professionals play in the identification of suspected adverse events.

Report Forms & Additional Information

FDA Drug Quality Reporting System	800-FDA-1088
Institute for Safe Medication Practices	215-956-9181
USP Drug Product Problem Reporting Program (in Maryland, call collect: 301-881-0256)	800-638-6725
USP Medication Error Reporting Program	800-23-ERROR
USP Practitioners' Reporting Network (an FDA MedWatch partner)	800-4-USP-PRN
Vaccine Adverse Events Reporting System (VAERS)	800-822-7967

References

[1] Kapit RM, Grabenstein JD. Adverse events after immunization: Reports & results. *Hosp Pharm* 1995;30:1031-2,1035-6,1038,1041.
[2] Chen RT, Rastogi SC, Mullen JR, et al. The Vaccine Adverse Event Reporting System (VAERS). *Vaccine* 1994;12:542-50.
[3] Bolger GR, Knapp DE, Reinstein PF, et al. FDA's drug quality reporting system. *Consult Pharm* 1992;7:28-31.
[4] Kessler DA. Introducing MedWatch: A new approach to reporting medication and device adverse effects and product problems. *JAMA* 1993;269:2765-8.
[5] Clayton EW, Hickson GB. Compensation under the National Childhood Vaccine Injury Act. *J Pediatr* 1990;116:508-13.
[6] Department of Health & Human Services. National Vaccine Injury Compensation Program revision of Vaccine Injury Table. *Fed Reg* 1995;60:7678-96.
[7] Grabenstein JD. Compensation for vaccine injury: Balancing society's need and personal risk. *Hosp Pharm* 1995;30:831-2,834-6.
[8] Landwirth J. Medical-legal aspects of immunization: Policy and practices. *Pediatr Clin N Amer* 1990;37:771-84.
[9] Fine PEM, Chen RT. Confounding in studies of adverse reactions to vaccines. *Am J Epidemiol* 1992;136:121-35.
[10] Neustadt RE, Fineberg HV. *The Epidemic That Never Was: Policy-Making & The Swine Flu Affair.* New York: Vintage Books, 1983.
[11] Silverstein AM. *Pure Politics & Impure Science: The Swine Flu Affair.* Baltimore: Johns Hopkins University Press, 1981.
[12] Langmuir AD, Bregman DJ, Kurland LT, et al. An epidemiologic and clinical evaluation of Guillain-Barré syndrome reported in association with the administration of swine influenza vaccines. *Am J Epidemiol* 1984;119:841-79.

ANNEX D

Hypersensitivities to Vaccine Components

Several recent review articles addressed many details about hypersensitivities to vaccine components, the diluents, adjuvants and excipients that go into vaccines; and issues of vaccine side effects and precautions.[1-3] This section presents the barest summary of those articles. Consult the full articles and other sources for details on these and other hypersensitivities.[1-4]

Background

Anaphylaxis is probably the most feared risk of immunization, but it is very rare. The risk is about one anaphylactic reaction for every 600,000 to 6.4 million doses of vaccine distributed. Because anaphylaxis often can be treated successfully, the risk of death from anaphylaxis is even more rare. A claim to hypersensitivity is not an automatic contraindication against immunization. First, confirm the diagnosis. Ask what event occurred that prompted the claim of allergy. Allergies in general do run in families, but family history is irrelevant to an individual's specific risk. Then, consider the patient's history in light of the following facts.

Egg Proteins

The viruses that go into measles, mumps, influenza and yellow-fever vaccines are grown in various forms of cultures involving hens' eggs. The long-standing rule has been that people who can eat eggs without alarm can be vaccinated with egg-based vaccines. Those who develop laryngeal edema, wheezing, nausea, anaphylaxis or related symptoms upon ingesting eggs warrant evaluation. This might include skin testing and escalating partial doses of vaccine. Hypersensitivities to feathers, chicken meat and other derivatives are irrelevant. If the person sneezes when exposed to feather pillows or gets an upset stomach from eating chicken meat, insufficient grounds exist to bar immunization.

In fact, people who are supposedly allergic to eggs rarely react to skin testing or measles-mumps-rubella (MMR) vaccine. Among 284 egg-allergic people, none had an adverse reaction to full-dose MMR vaccine.[5] Of 1209 people with positive skin-test reactions to egg, all received MMR vaccine without adverse event. Only two of the 1227 egg-allergic people vaccinated with MMR had any symptoms consistent with anaphylaxis. At least 38 cases of anaphylactic reactions to measles or MMR vaccines in people without allergy to eggs have been reported. While people do react severely to MMR in extraordinarily rare cases, egg hypersensitivity does little to predict it.

The ACIP is reevaluating its long-standing recommendation for skin testing people with severe egg hypersensitivities.[3,6] Canadian experts have already decided to remove egg allergy as a contraindication to MMR immunization.[7-8]

Thimerosal

Thimerosal is a mercurial preservative added to many immunologic drugs. Thimerosal caused false-positive tuberculin reactions until it was removed from formulations. Thimerosal is most troublesome in drugs applied to the skin or eyes. No severe or life-threatening systemic reactions to parenteral use of thimerosal have been reported, although urticaria and other dermatologic reactions have rarely been associated with thimerosal- containing vaccines. Delayed hypersensitivity to thimerosal is not grounds for deferring parenteral immunization with a drug containing thimerosal. This includes people who avoid thimerosal in contact-lens solutions. The vaccine's value will almost always outweigh this miniscule risk.

Neomycin

Neomycin is used to prevent the growth of adventitious bacteria in industrial viral cultures. Most neomycin hypersensitivity manifests as contact dermatitis or delayed hypersensitivity. Consequently, the likelihood of an anaphylactoid reaction from a parenteral dose of neomycin is exceptionally remote. Neomycin skin tests may introduce several-fold higher doses of neomycin into the body than the vaccine itself: 100 to 1000 mcg vs 25 mcg. As a result, testing holds little value. In summary, the vaccines' value almost always outweighs the risk of delayed neomycin hypersensitivity.

Gelatin

Gelatin is added as a stabilizer or filler in several vaccines. A few cases of anaphylaxis were reported in Europe after infusion of plasma volume expanders consisting of modified gelatin. Some anaphylactic reactions to MMR vaccine have been attributed to gelatin stabilizers based on antibody tests and skin tests. These people also may develop allergic reactions upon ingesting gelatin in food. The risk of gelatin causing anaphylaxis after immunization is extremely rare.

Aluminum

Aluminum compounds are added as adjuvants to several vaccines. Subcutaneous nodules occur in some people injected with vaccines containing aluminum adjuvants. These nodules typically disappear spontaneously within a few weeks. More rarely, nodules persist for up to a year.

Lactose

Lactose is included as a filler in several vaccines. Lactose intolerance is a deficiency of the intestinal enzyme lactase. Lactose intolerance causes cramps, diarrhea, distension and flatulence. Parenteral administration has not been associated with lactose intolerance. Immunologic drugs containing lactose are unlikely to cause problems because they contain only 2 to 180 mg lactose per dose, rather than the 3 to $>$ 5 g levels expected to exacerbate symptoms of lactase deficiency.

Monosodium Glutamate

Monosodium glutamate (MSG) acts as a stabilizer in several vaccines. MSG is associated with "Chinese-restaurant syndrome," involving warmth, chest tightness, sweating, nausea, numbness and tingling of the face, neck, upper chest, shoulders and upper arms in large oral doses. No adverse reactions to MSG in vaccines have been published in the professional literature. This may be because the pharmaceutical dose is several-fold less than the dose associated with a meal. MSG sensitivity is essentially irrelevant to administration of immunologic drugs.

Sulfites

Sulfites (eg, sodium metabisulfite) are antioxidants used as drug stabilizers. Sulfites preserve the integrity of the active ingredient under adverse conditions. Sulfites are added to at least one vaccine and to most formulations of epinephrine. Large oral doses of sulfites can cause dyspnea, wheezing, urticaria, diarrhea, vomiting, cramps and dizziness. In severe cases, systemic respiratory or circulatory collapse and CNS depression can occur. Most adverse events occur after oral exposure, although symptoms occasionally occur after parenteral administration. Regardless of a person's prior sensitivity to sulfites, do not withhold medications containing sulfites in life-threatening emergencies. Standard doses of epinephrine contain less sulfite than doses that typically provoke positive challenge tests.

Synthesis

Although rates of anaphylaxis after immunization are extraordinarily rare, the risk is > 0. Immunize only in settings where anaphylactic or other unexpected reactions can be managed adequately. This means having the proper emergency supplies and adequately trained personnel. Emergency responses are discussed in chapter 6 on "Immunization Administration."

When preparing to vaccinate someone, ask about that person's history of previous adverse reactions to drugs and foods. Ask for the names of offending agents, the type of reaction experienced and how long ago it was. Be wary of inappropriate contraindications.

Of the compounds discussed above, most cause adverse effects rarely; The main exception, given our present state of knowledge, involves severe allergies to eggs, gelatin or neomycin.

Prior adverse personal experience after immunization may validly contraindicate future doses, but such cases are extraordinarily rare. If allergy cannot be ruled out but the vaccine is indicated, the next step may be skin testing or desensitization. While usually safe, informed consent from the patient to skin testing or desensitization is reasonable. Always consider the risk-benefit ratio, and decide whether or not desensitization risks outweigh the benefits of immunity and avoiding the risks of the disease.

References

[1] Grabenstein JD. Clinical management of hypersensitivities to vaccine components. *Hosp Pharm* 1997;32:77-8,81-4,87.
[2] Grabenstein JD. Immunologic necessities: Diluents, adjuvants, & excipients. *Hosp Pharm* 1996;31:1387-8,1390,1392,1397-8,1401.
[3] Advisory Committee on Immunization Practices. Update: Vaccine side effects, adverse reactions, contraindications, and precautions. *MMWR* 1996;45(RR-12):1-35. Errata 1997;46:227.
[4] Grabenstein JD. *ImmunoFacts: Vaccines & Immunologic Drugs*. St. Louis: Facts and Comparisons, Inc., May 1997.
[5] James JM, Burks AW, Roberson PK, et al. Safe administration of the measles vaccine to children allergic to eggs. *N Engl J Med* 1995;332:1262-6.
[6] Murphy KR, Strunk RC. Safe administration of influenza vaccine in asthmatic children hypersensitive to egg proteins. *J Pediatr* 1985;106:931-3.
[7] Canadian National Advisory Committee on Immunizations. *Canadian Immunization Guide,* 4th ed. Ottawa: Ministry of National Health & Welfare, 1993.
[8] Canadian National Advisory Committee on Immunization. MMR vaccine and anaphylactic hypersensitivity to egg or egg-related antigens. *Can Comm Dis Rep* 1996;22:113-5.

INDEX

A

Active Listening, 48
Active vs Passive Immunity, 30
Adenovirus vaccine tablets, 83
Administration Guidelines, 77
Administrative Issues, 107
Adolescent Immunization Checklist, 55
Adrenalin, 84
Adverse drug experience reports, 175
Advocacy Ideas, 163
Age, advancing, 67
AIDS, Vaccine Recommendations for People with, 71, 73
Allergic Hypersensitivity, 84
Aluminum, 180
Ana-Kit, 86
Anaphylaxis management, 83
Annotated Screening Form for Vaccines, 95
Anti-rabies serum, 30
Assessment and Feedback, 46
Asthma, 11, 25
Azathioprine, 11

B

BCG vaccine, 71
Billing Codes, 115
Booster vs Primary Responses, 31
Bordetella pertussis, 17
Breast-feeding, 67
Breath-holding, 88

C

Catalogs, product, 169
CDC Fax Information Service, 172
Centers for Disease Control, 172
Cellular vs Humoral Immunity, 29
Chickenpox - See Varicella
"Childhood" Diseases, 13
Cholera vaccine, 72
Choosing a Route, 79
Circulating vs Local Antibodies, 31
Clinic Immunization Record, 102
Clostridium tetani, 16, 32
CMV - see Cytomegalovirus
Community Catalysts, 160
Community Collaboration and Leadership, 166
Compensation for Immunizing, 108
Compensation for Vaccine Injury, 128
Compounding Dilutions, 37
Confirmation, 60
Congenital rubella syndrome, 14
Consent and Education, 57
Consent Forms, 59
Contraindications, 52
Corynebacterium diphtheriae, 16, 32
Cost-effectiveness, 5
Counseling Techniques, 47
Customizing Immunization Plans, 65

D

Decision-Making, 54
Delayed Hypersensitivity, 179
Deliver the Dose, 78
Diagnoses Warranting Immunization, 25
Differential Utilization, 38
Digoxin Immune Fab, 11
Diluents, 37
Dilution Compounding, 37
Diphenhydramine Doses, 85
Diphtheria, 16, 20
Diphtheria and tetanus toxoids (adult), 16, 72
Diphtheria and tetanus toxoids (pediatric), 16, 72
Disease vs Infection, 31
Diseases and Diagnoses of People Needing Vaccines, 25
Diseases Warranting Immunization, 11, 25
Documentation, Immunization, 93
Drug Interactions, 34
Drug Product Problem Reporting Program, 177
Drug Quality Reporting System, 176
Drugs Indicative of Diseases Warranting Immunizations, 26
DT - see Diphtheria and tetanus toxoids (pediatric)
DTP - see Diphtheria and tetanus toxoids with pertussis vaccine

E

Education and Consent, 57
Egg-hypersensitivity assessment, 179
Emergency Plans, 83
Engerix-B, 12
EpiEZPen Jr., 86
EpiEZPen, 86
Epinephrine, 84
Epinephrine Comparisons, 86
Epinephrine Doses, 85
EpiPen Jr., 85, 86
EpiPen, 83, 86

F

Facility Design, 107
Fainting, 87
Filing a Medicare Reimbursement Claim, 109
Finding Those Who Need Vaccines, 43
Food & Drug Administration, 173
Form, Immunization-Need Screening, 95
Form, Informed Consent, 59, 103

G

Gelatin, 180
General Rule – Contraindications and Precautions, 52
Getting Started, 159
Glycerin, 37
Grass-Roots Coalitions, 167

H

Haemophilus influenzae type b, 19, 33, 72
Haemophilus influenzae type b polysaccharide vaccine, 19, 33
Handling and administration, 77
HBIG - see Hepatitis B immune globulin
HCPCS Codes, 110
Hepatitis A, 72
Hepatitis A vaccine, 36
Hepatitis B, 11, 20, 72
Hepatitis B immune globulin, 12
Hepatitis B vaccine, 12, 30
Heptavax-B, 12, 30
Hib - see *Haemophilus influenzae* type b vaccine
HIV, Vaccine Recommendations for People Infected with, 71
How To Motivate Vaccine Candidates, 45
How Vaccines and Antibodies Work, 29
Human immunodeficiency virus, 71
Human vs Animal Antibodies, 33
Humoral vs Cellular Immunity, 29
Hydroxyurea, 11
Hymenoptera venoms, 37
Hyperimmune vs Standard Antibodies, 35
Hypersensitivities to Vaccine Components, 179
Hypersensitivity Categories, 179
Hyperventilation, 87

I

IMIG - see Immune globulin intramuscular
Immune Globulin, intramuscular, 36
Immune Globulin, intravenous, 36
Immune plasmas, 36
Immunization Administration, 77
Immunization Documentation, 102
Immunization Needs, International Travel, 67
Immunocompromised people, 69
Immunodeficiency, 69
Immunologic Drug Interactions, 34
Immunosuppressants, 34
Inappropriate Contraindications, 50
Infection vs Disease, 31
Influenza, 8, 20, 72
Influenza A and B vaccine, 8
Informed-Consent Documents, 59, 103
Injection site, 79
Injury Compensation Program, Vaccine, 131
Interactions of Immunologic Drugs, 34
International Travel Recommendations, 67
Interviewing People About Immunizations, 46
Interviewing Techniques, 47
Intradermal Injection, 82
Intramuscular Injection, 79
Introduction: Focus on Prevention, 1
IPV - see Poliovirus vaccine, inactivated
Issues of Age, 67
IVIG - see Immune Globulin intravenous

K

Key questions to ask patients, 49
Key questions to help advocates get started, 159
Killed vs Live Vaccines, 32

L

Lactation, 67
Lactose, 180
Legal and Liability Issues, 124, 150
Liability, 124
Live vs Killed Vaccines, 32
Local vs Circulating Antibodies, 31
Lost Records, 104

M

Making Vaccine Decisions, 43
Management Issues, 107
Marketing Issues, 107
Measles, 13, 20
Measles vaccine, 13
Measles-mumps-rubella vaccine, 14
Medicare Reimbursement, 109
Medication Error Reporting Program, 185
Medications and Diseases as Indicators, 11
Medications of People Needing Vaccines, 26
Medicine's Role in Immunization Delivery, 153
MedWatch, 185
Memory and Recall, 93
Meningococcal vaccine A/C/Y/W-135, 72
Misconceptions about Contraindications, 50
MMR - see Measles-mumps-rubella vaccine
Model of Health Behavior, 45
Monosodium glutamate, 181
Motivation, 45
Mumps, 14, 29
Mumps skin test antigen, 29
Mumps vaccine, 14, 29

N

National Childhood Vaccine Injury Act, 99
Neomycin, 180
Nursing's Role in Immunization Delivery, 147

O

Obtaining Compensation, 108
Opportunities, 60
OPV - see Poliovirus vaccine, oral
Oral Administration, 83
Other Management Issues, 107
Other Urgent Situations, 88
Outcome vs Process, 40

P

Partners in Immunization Advocacy, 172
Passive vs Active Immunity,
Penicillamine, 26
Pertussis, 17
Pertussis vaccine, 17
Pharmacy's Role in Immunization Delivery, 135
Phenol-saline, 37
Plague vaccine, 72

Pneumococcal Disease, 9, 72
Pneumococcal polysaccharide vaccine, 10
Pneumonia, Pneumococcal, 10, 20
Policy Making, 38
Poliomyelitis, 18
Poliovirus vaccine, live, oral, trivalent, 18, 32, 71
Poliovirus vaccine inactivated, 19, 32
Polysaccharide vs Protein Vaccines, 33
Power of Suggestion, 59
PPD - see Tuberculin, purified protein derivative
Precautions, 52
Pregnancy, 65
Prepare the Dose, 77
Prepare the Patient, 77
Prescription Drugs, 26
Preservatives, 37, 180
Primary vs Booster Responses, 31
Print Resources, 169
Process vs Outcome, 40
Product Catalogs, 174
Production Methods, 36
Protein vs Polysaccharide Vaccines, 33

Q

Questions to ask patients, 47

R

Rabies immune globulin, 30, 33
Rabies vaccine, 30
Recall and Reminder Systems, 60
Recombivax-HB, 12
Recommendations for International Travel, 67
Records, Immunization, 102
Reimbursement, Medicare, 109
Relative Cost-effectiveness, 5
Reminder and Recall Systems, 60
Resources Available, 169
Respiratory Obstructions, 88
Response to a Systemic Reaction, 84
Reye's syndrome, 2
RIG - see Rabies immune globulin
Roster Billing, 120
Route and site, 79
Rubella, 14
Rubella vaccine, 15

S

Sabin poliovirus vaccine, 32
Safety of Immunizing HIV-Infected People, 73
Salk poliovirus vaccine, 32
Science of Vaccinology, 29
Screening for Vaccine Needs, 49
Screening Methods, 49
Seizures, 88
Sodium chloride diluent, 37
Solutions vs Suspensions, 35
Sources of Additional Information, 170
Special Situations, 65
Standard Vaccine Advice Based on Age, 90
Standard vs Hyperimmune Antibodies, 35
State and Selected Local Health Departments, 170
State Immunization Program Managers, 170
Streptococcus pneumoniae, 9
Subcutaneous Injection, 81
Subunit vs Whole Vaccines, 34
Sulfites, 181
Suspensions vs Solutions, 35

T

Tetanus, 16, 20
Tetanus and diphtheria toxoids (adult), 72
Tetanus and diphtheria toxoids (pediatric), 72
Tetanus antitoxin, 17
Thimerosal, 37, 180
Timing and Spacing of Vaccines, 56
Timing in Relation to Antibodies, 56
Too Many Deaths, Too Much Disease, 7
Toxoids vs Vaccines, 32
Typhoid fever, 32

U

Underlying Disease, 68
Upper Respiratory Obstructions, 88

V

Vaccine Adverse Event Reporting System (VAERS), 175
Vaccine Advice for People Infected with HIV, 71
Vaccine Indications, Based on Age, 89
Vaccine Injury Compensation Program, 131
Vaccine Injury Table, 133
Vaccine Records for Clinicians, 94
Vaccine Records for Patients, 103
Vaccine Schedules, 54
Vaccine-Preventable Infections, 7
Vaccines Are Drugs, 29
Vaccines vs Toxoids, 32
VAERS, 175
Varicella, 15, 20
Varicella vaccine, 15, 71
Varicella-zoster immune globulin, 15
VIG - see Vaccinia immune globulin
Visit Sketches, 89
VZIG - see Varicella-zoster immune globulin

W

Waste disposal, 107
Weakened Immune Systems, 68
Whole vs Subunit Vaccines, 34
Whooping cough, 17

Y

Yellow-fever vaccine, 71

Z

Zidovudine, 11
Zoster, 15